PAIN, PAIN GO AWAY

How Reconstructive Therapy Eliminates Backache, Carpal Tunnel Syndrome, Knee Pain, Migraine, Headache, Sciatica, Arthritis, Tendonitis, Fibrositis, Temporomandibular Joint Syndrome, Failed Orthopedic Surgery, Failed Neurosurgery, and Other Disabilities from Injured Tendons, Unstable Ligaments and Inflamed Joints, Regardless of the Sufferer's Age or Duration of His or Her Pain Problem

by

William J. Faber, D.O.
Practicing Doctor of Osteopathic Medicine
Founder and Medical Director
Milwaukee Pain Clinic And Metabolic Research Center
Milwaukee, Wisconsin

and

Morton Walker, D.P.M.
Medical Journalist and Editorial Director
Freelance Communications
Stamford, Connecticut

Illustrations by
Richard Marvin Voigt
Brookfield, Wisconsin

Published by
ISHI PRESS INTERNATIONAL
76 Bonaventura Drive
San Jose, CA 95134
U.S.A.

Available in Europe from
ISHI INTERNATIONAL, LTD.
P.O. Box 3288
London NW5 1RQ, U.K.

First printing March 1990
Second printing September 1990
Third printing September 1991
Fourth printing March 1992
Fifth printing April 1993
Sixth printing October 1993
Seventh printing June 1994
Eighth printing January 1995

Printed in U.S.A.

Dedication

To those seeking relief and have not been able to find it.

To Randy, the boy I used to know.

Disclaimer

This book has been written and published strictly for informational purposes. In no way should it be used as a substitute for your own physician's advice.

While William J. Faber, D.O. and Morton Walker, D. P. M., are collaborating here as co-authors, Dr. Faber is the physician expert on reconstructive therapy and Dr. Walker is the medical journalist reporting on such health care information.

You should not consider educational material in this book to be the practice of medicine, although almost all the statements have come from the files, publications, and personal interviews of informed physicians who diagnose and treat chronic joint, tendon, and ligament pain and their patients who have suffered from these difficulties. Moreover, lecture presentations, audiotapes, published case reports, medical documentation of patient trials, anecdotes, testimonials, patient histories — all from physicians experienced in the application of joint reconstruction techniques — have been utilized to educate our readers.

The successes with joint pain correction are facts reported from the clinical experiences of osteopathic and allopathic physicians over the last sixty-five years.

If you, as a potential user of knowledge received from these pages, require opinions, diagnoses, treatments, therapeutic advice, correction of your lifestyle, or any other aid relating to your health, it is recommended that you consult a medical expert on reconstructive therapy. A list of such therapeutic experts is appended to this book.

These statements are to be considered disclaimers of responsibility for anything published here. The co-authors are providing the information in this book with the understanding that you may act on it at your own risk and also with full knowledge that health professionals should first be consulted and that their specific advice for you should be considered before accepting anything read here.

All physicians, surgeons, and other health professionals are informed that joint reconstruction therapy is a serious procedure which should not be employed without specific preceptorship training. Adverse results, including death, have been reported by its incorrect application. This book is not intended for a health professional's training but only for medical consumer education.

Table of Contents

Foreword

It is a pleasure to write a foreword for this well-written, easily read, and accurately presented new book, *Pain, Pain Go Away*, by William J. Faber, D.O. and Morton Walker, D.P.M. The two authors take a subject that ordinarily is difficult to understand and make it fully comprehensible.

This book is aptly titled. My experience with reconstructive therapy has been that, when indicated, it is exceedingly satisfactory and rewarding for my patients. I know that the human body most often heals itself, but occasionally it welcomes a helping hand. Reconstructive therapy offers that hand.

My own chiropractic specialty·is Applied Kinesiolgy, yet there have been quite a few times when I refer patients for reconstructive therapy. Dr. Hackett first introduced me to the joint-reconstruction concepts that my good friend Dr. Bill Faber now so competently administers. In this text, he and his coauthor precisely describe the treatment for all types of patients with joint, tendon, and/or ligamentous problems.

Chronic joint pain is the nemesis of the world's population. It is responsible for the American public alone spending over $5.2 billion a year for prescription drugs and another $2.2 billion for non-prescription drugs. Still, two-thirds of them would be unnecessary, if people would just look at some of the holistic concepts available in modern practice today. Instead of merely masking pain, the mechanical causes of pain can be corrected.

The alternative treatment method for chronic joint pain presented by the authors is not intended as a panacea for all health problems. Rather, reconstructive therapy is directed toward the reduction of health-care costs, prevention of needless surgery, avoidance of useless medication, and elimination of dangers from receiving such drugs and surgery.

The purpose of *Pain, Pain Go Away*, then is to educate the medical consumer about a safe, simple, easy-to-receive technique that has been proven effective repeatedly during the last forty years and successfully administered to tens of thousands of those who had formerly suffered with joint, tendon, and/or ligament troubles.

Understanding the reconstructive therapeutic approach is not at all difficult. You will learn of it here, perhaps even before your doctor does. Do that health professional a favor and present this text to him or her as a gift. Give it to your attorney, worker's compensation administrator, judge, insurance company, your social worker, too. They are just a few of the people who make important decisions, but who need to be educated about what can be done for chronic joint pain.

Dr. Walker has turned Dr. Faber's scientific information into comprehensible and comprehensive prose. Dr. Faber is an expert when it comes to relieving a patient's chronic joint pain. The ilustrations by Richard Marvin Voigt depicting our normal and dysfunctional joints are fabulously drawn. Mr. Voigt has produced artistic renditions that are faithful to the body's normal anatomy, to the pathology of disrepair, and to the overall therapeutic approach of reconstructive therapy. Congratulations to these three artist/scientists for a completed book that is extremely well done. It will educate millions about chronic joint pain relief!

George J. Goodheart, Jr. D.C.,
Discover and Developer of Applied Kinesilogy
Grosse Pointe Woods, Michigan
October 2, 1989

Preface

Of all the reasons for an individual's quality of life deteriorating, chronic joint pain is the most common.

Any day of the year, one American in five suffers from some form of crippling symptoms of persistent, deep-seated, and recurring articular agony. Joint troubles have reached epidemic proportions and are directly responsible for reducing this country's gross national product by $80 billion a year.

In underdeveloped, developing, and industrialized countries alike, chronic pain from injured tendons, unstable ligaments, and inflamed joints produce more financial loss, social burden, physical disability, emotional upset, and mental suffering than all other degenerative disorders and infectious diseases, combined.

For its physician-readers, for example, the April 22, 1987 issue of *Medical Tribune* reported that in the United States each year, the public spends over $20 billion on professional health care just for backache arising from inflamed intervertebral joints. "Backache costs another $40 billion annually in workman's compensation, legal fees, social security, and disability payments," said Tom Mayer, M.D., Assistant Clinical Professor of Orthopedic Surgery at the University of Texas Health Science Center at Dallas. Vert Mooney, M.D., chairman of Dr. Mayer's department, confirms that backache, affecting some 15 million Americans each year, taxes the health care system more than the three major health disablers: coronary artery disease, high blood pressure, or diabetes.

Moreover, the National Center for Health Statistics reports that while backache is one of the leading reasons people are forced to spend time in hospitals, hip injuries and their chronic residual symptoms among the elderly lead to the longest stays. According to the Medicare Division of the U.S. Social Security Administration, hip trauma with resultant chronic hip joint pain is the most prevalent musculoskeletal difficulty experienced by Americans over age sixty-five.

The director of Boston's Robert B. Bringham Multipurpose Arthritis Center, Matthew H. Liang, M.D., estimates that the cost of arthritis alone in the United States is $16 billion annually in lost or reduced productivity, forfeited wages, direct health costs, and disability payments.

Backache, hip trauma, and arthritis are only a few of the chronic joint pain troublemakers. There also are spondylolisthesis, whiplash, carpal tunnel syndrome, migraine headaches, knee problems, foot faults, shoulder dislocations, wrecked wrists, pain after orthopedic surgery, and a great deal more. Many people are permanently disabled from chronic joint pain of one kind or another. For instance, in another report, the Social Security Administration said that in 1986 it paid out permanent disability benefits for chronic joint pain alone to six million people. In 1988, over seven million pensioners and other disabled persons received compensation for this one type of problem.

Disability payments for chronic joint pain were the total support moneys on which all of these Americans survived. It was pain from their joint disorders that prevented them in any other way from earning subsistence income.

Pain among the populace is beneficial to certain drug companies. Chronicity brings them big financial rewards. The trade magazine of the pharmaceutical industry, *Medical Advertising News*, told subscribers in its April 1, 1987 issue that as in prior years the best-selling prescription pharmaceuticals of 1986 were pain-killers. The same types of drugs were popular the next year, as well — and then the next. Manufactured by McNeil Consumer Products Company, Tylenol with Codeine™ has led the field by ranking first in product sales for six consecutive years. Chronic joint pain has repeatedly proven itself to be the great human disabler — a real money-maker — and the generic drug in Tylenol™, acetaminophen, is far surpassing aspirin in annual pain-killer sales.

The Need to Educate Consumers about Chronic Joint Pain

Around the world, the medical profession and health care systems have grown more aware of the gigantic dimension of chronic pain problems. Consequently, they have explored new techniques for proper evaluation, classification, and treatment of them. Information evolves, finds publication in the medical literature, and eventually gets applied clinically for patient relief. However, such information quite often is highly scientific and fails to reach the general public. The person who suffers with symptoms of long duration usually is left with little knowledge, unless it is geared to 'the miracles' of a new drug approach. Such public relations news most often is financed by the pharmaceutical manufacturers who are offering the 'miracle' drugs for sale. Consumers get educated only about the aspect of pain relief that will line the pockets of those drug companies that want to popularize drug products for pain.

Information that you find here is different. It has no prescriptions or over-the-counter remedies to pitch. Instead, our message is intended to shorten the communication gap for people victimized by chronic joint pain. The subject of our book's discussion, reconstructive therapy, effectively treats nearly all tendon, ligament, and joint problems by permanently strengthening injured areas. The main side effect of tendon, ligament, and joint reconstruction is the elimination of pain.

Our text dedicates itself to enlightening those who have vested interests in knowing more: pain sufferers, primary care physicians, third-party health cost compensators, health insurance companies, worker's compensation administrators, lawyers, judges, government health officials, Social Security administrators, social and welfare agency administrators, lawmakers in state and federal governments, employers, athletic team trainers and their athletes, plus others advising about human incapacity from pain in the musculoskeletal system.

Plenty of books have been published about individual joint problems such as fascitis, bunions and other foot trouble, arthritis, backache, knee trouble, sports injuries, migraine headache, shoulder dislocation, and pain in general, but *Pain, Pain Go Away* is devoted specifically to the cause and correction of dysfunction arising from unstable joints. Such instability results from degenerative disease, overly lax ligaments, torn tendons, ruptured discs, and/or crushed cartilage. Never before has there been a complete source of information about the causative factors and permanent corrective procedures for chronic pain in the joints, tendons, and ligaments.

The co-authors' research for this book has been concerned with recurrent or ever present joint pain and the true medical breakthrough that eliminates it. We describe treatment, relief, and cure for painful joint handicaps of many types — a procedure developed, tested, utilized, and verified by over 250 American, Canadian, Australian, and European medical doctors and osteopathic physicians. Osteopaths are the chief health professional exponents of this correction. Clinicians, turned researchers, have joined together in a scholarly organization, the American Osteopathic Academy of Sclerotherapy, an official affiliate of the American Osteopathic Association. In a paper published in the July 18, 1987 issue of the prestigious British medical journal *The Lancet*, Milne J. Ongley, M.D., Robert G. Klein, M.D., Thomas A. Dorman, M.D., Bjorn C. Eek, M.D., and Lawrence J. Hubert, M.D. of the Department of Rheumatology, Sansum Medical Clinic of Santa Barbara, California affirmed that reconstructive therapy has an 88 percent rate of success for the elimination of chronic low back pain, and it was accomplished with just six series of proliferant injections. Other published medical journal papers written by many internationally acclaimed doctor/researchers say the same for various parts of the body. William Kubitschek, D.O. of San Marcos, California estimates that 600,000 people worldwide have taken reconstructive therapeutic injections. Dr. Kubitschek, a reconstructive therapist, is quoted as stating that approximately 450,000 North Americans, 66,000 Australians and New Zealanders, 51,000 Europeans, and others are estimated to have been treated to date. They were formerly suffering from the agony of chronic joint discomfort but are not pain victims any longer.

You are about to learn how a person in constant agony, regardless of how long he or she has suffered, can be helped by means of an established but little known treatment technique first described in the medical literature approximately sixty years ago. Formerly called "sclerotherapy," and then labeled "prolotherapy" by George S. Hackett, M.D., the grandfather of modern concepts for this treatment and consulting surgeon at Mercy Hospital in Canton, Ohio. "Proliferative therapy" was its next designation. Physicians now have finally adopted the clearer and more descriptive names for this procedure of "reconstructive therapy" or "joint, ligament, and tendon reconstruction."

No matter what label the treatment is given, *Pain, Pain Go Away* tells medical consumers how to permanently rid themselves of pain arising from nearly any kind of damaged joint, ligament, and tendon. As a result of the effectiveness of reconstructive therapy, typical musculoskeletal lesions that may be permanently corrected are: bunions, heel difficulties, finger dysfunctions, patellar problems, migraine headache, neck pain, chronic shoulder dislocation, rotator cuff tears, generalized back weakness, herniated disks, mid-level backache, low back pain, compression fractures of the vertebrae, ankylosing spondylitis, spondylolisthesis, fibrositis, fascitis, tendonitis, pain after severe injury, pain after stroke, temporomandibular joint (TMJ) syndrome, post-orthopedic surgery pain, dysfunctional hip joint, chronic and acute knee disability, ankle weakness, tennis leg, tennis elbow, wrist pain, carpal-tunnel syndrome, and most forms of arthritis, especially the type derived from wear and tear (osteoarthritis), and more disabilities. Reconstructive therapy is often a medical alternative to orthopedic surgery, hand surgery, podiatric surgery, and other traditional techniques of musculo-skeletal repair.

We are endeavoring to give new insight into the traditional medical methods of diagnosis and/or treatment of joint pain — procedures that fail because they are based on incorrect concepts of joint pathology. Such erroneous procedures include the use of exercise, cortisone injections, physical therapy, laminectomy, other surgeries designed to remove cartilage or disks, and pain-killers that don't work. These are therapeutic falsehoods which are thought of as standards of care, but in too many instances just fail the patient altogether, leaving millions to seek their own means of relief.

While every individual case history presented by us is true and about a real person, pseudonyms are employed because of requirements of many of the State Medical Societies. The information in this book comes from literature searches and other research done by co- author Morton Walker, D.P.M. and from patient interviews he conducted. The case reports, patient contacts, and the scientific basis for joint pain elimination have been supplied by William Faber, D.O. and his colleagues at the American Osteopathic Academy of Sclerotherapy, the American Association of Orthopaedic Medicine, the American Academy of Neurologic and Orthopaedic Surgeons, and the Canadian Association of Orthopedic Medicine. These are the doctors who have taken training in the techniques of joint reconstruction, participate in preceptorships, and attend seminars on the subject so as to exchange new information with each other.

We have used the artistic talent of professional medical illustrator Richard Marvin Voigt of Milwaukee for the medical illustrations depicted in this book. It is anticipated that the drawings and our text will be useful to you and/or your loved ones so as to eliminate joint, tendon, and ligament disabilities from your lives. Our desires and expectations are that return to normal joint function and complete comfort in daily activities will be the experience of every reader who takes this book's information seriously and acts upon it, according to his or her belief and physical need.

William J. Faber, D.O., S.C., Medical Director
Milwaukee Pain Clinic and Metabolic Research Center
Milwaukee, Wisconsin

and

Morton B. Walker, D.P.M., Medical Journalist
and Editorial Director
FREELANCE COMMUNICATIONS
Stamford, Connecticut

January 2, 1990

Chapter One

Do You or Your Loved Ones Have Chronic Joint Pain?

Would you be interested in knowing of a safe, effective, tested, legal, nonsurgical treatment that provides increased endurance and function to joints, tendons, and ligaments with its main side effect being the elimination of pain?

Would you want to take treatment that can increase a joint's mobility and strength and stop its pain regardless of how many years stiffness, weakness, and discomfort have existed?

Would you be anxious for treatment that repairs weakened or torn body parts permanently by use of natural healing mechanisms?

Would you prefer this procedure to other less effective medical techniques that are directed against relieving symptoms but not correcting disease?

Would you like to avoid hazardous health care methods such as knee surgery, laminectomy, hip replacement, chymopapaine injections, cortisone injections, and prescriptions for pain killers or oral cortisone that often fail or leave you with awful side effects?

Would you want your family physician to know all about this effective treatment and set you to following a lifestyle that could add pain-free years to the time you have to live?

Would you be dubious if an informed person told you that some orthopedic surgeons and other high-priced practitioners did not have any knowledge of this trustworthy correction and might refuse to prescribe it even if they did?

Would you be surprised to learn that the technique's application takes much skill and requires thorough knowledge of musculoskeletal anatomy and physiology, but is not taught in medical schools or residency training?

If you or your loved one needed such a treatment, would you feel frustration at not being informed of its existence when your physician presented the ways and means to overcome your chronic joint pain problem? This is the real situation for millions of people attempting to control their pain.

Suppose you and others who love her see the prolonged suffering felt by your elderly mother from a pain in her right hip joint. It never lets up. She lives in a nursing home, and the general practitioner called in diagnoses her trouble as bursitis. But when it comes to offering treatment, he just shrugs his shoulders and says, "Give her two aspirin every four hours." Repeated doses of aspirin offer no relief at all and irritate her hiatal hernia as well, so the aspirin is discontinued.

Observing your mother's continued inability to function — not even able to go to the toilet without assistance — you bring her to a neurologist. He says that the diagnosis of bursitis is wrong; rather, she is the victim of neuropathy. He tells you in private, "There's nothing to be done for an 84-year-old neuropathy patient like your mother. Just give her nursing care. Do what's possible to keep her comfortable. I'll write a prescription for Tylenol with Codeine™. Call me if refills are needed."

This was the situation for Anna Columbine, the mother of Rose O'Keefe of Garden City, Kansas. Mrs. O'Keefe's family physician is V.A. Leopold, D.O., also of Garden City. Dr. Leopold, still in active practice and engaged with osteopathic medicine for sixty-four years, is ten years older even than Mrs. Columbine.

At Mrs. O'Keefe's request, the osteopathic physician examined her mother on December 10, 1984. Based on X-ray, laboratory, and clinical examinations that showed no arthritis in the hip, no bursitis, and no particularly significant signs or symptoms of neuropathy, Dr. Leopold decided that a sprained ligament around the femoral joint was the source of his new patient's pain.

When he put pressure over the femur (thigh bone), Mrs. Columbine "just about jumped off the examination table," he wrote to us. Dr. Leopold also found a short left limb and subluxation (dislocation) of the left posterior sacroiliac which he corrected by osteopathic manipulation. This subluxation was a partial dislocation at the rear of the junction where the sacrum joins the ilium. The bones were misaligned but still in contact.

Dr. Leopold gave Mrs. Columbine reconstructive therapy, injecting the corrective solution over and around the femoral joint and as far as possible around its encompassing ligament. He reports, "She had been walking with a walker, and now — within a few days — she began walking without any help at all. The pain was practically relieved entirely. I repeated this treatment about two weeks later on January 2, 1985. One more injection took away any traces of the hip pain. The joint was stabilized. This joint and ligament reconstruction has corrected her condition until this day [July 6, 1989]. She was discharged from the nursing home and has been active at home ever since."

Scott Drake, a twenty-nine-year-old iron worker from Atlanta, Georgia, was seeing his life come apart because of an injury he sustained while playing touch football six months earlier. Scott is a macho-type individual, six-foot, two-inches tall, and 185 pounds. He has shoulders like a line backer, thighs the circumference of small tree trunks, and very well-developed biceps from lifting weights. Body building is his hobby. Along with his brawn, however, Scott Drake has sandy-colored hair, manly features, and a ready wit and boyish smile. His attributes won him one of the prettiest girls in Atlanta to be his wife.

Scott's touch football injury had his right ankle badly swollen and it remained weakened — giving out on him spontaneously even half a year after the accident. If he walked on an uneven surface, his ankle would cave in and produce a new flare-up of swelling and pain, just the way it behaved when the injury occurred. This was a hazardous condition to be in because of the young man's occupation. After ten years with the union, Scott had earned his position of journeyman iron worker. The wages were excellent. When he worked thirty stories in the air on the skeletons of buildings attaching steel beams with hot rivets, he brought home nearly $24 an hour, after taxes. Now, with a right ankle that he was unsure of, he was afraid to go up on the catwalks. Scott lacked confidence in his ability to balance on the 30-story-high beams.

He and his pretty wife were raising two small children. He had a house with a manageable mortgage and car payments. But for six months he felt unable to work. His ankle throbbed, and he was afraid to put his life on the line. Trying to do his usual work had him feeling morose. The man's savings were being eaten up, and in thirty days his unemployment checks would run out. He realized that he had to do something fast to recover.

His visit to a well-known orthopedic surgeon got him a diagnosis and treatment recommendation. The orthopedist told him that a surgical fusion would stabilize his ankle so that it would not cave in. Scott then asked about movement of the ankle. Motion and activity are essential to an iron worker's ability to perform on the job.

The surgeon said that to stabilize the ankle with a fusion,

4

much of the motion must be sacrificed. "That's what a fusion is for, to restrict motion between the foot and the leg at the ankle," he explained. "You can't have your cake and eat it too."

It was clear to Scott that surgery wasn't going to let him follow his trade as an iron worker, because trying to climb, kneel, and balance with a fused ankle just wouldn't be good enough. It could be the death of him. Ankle fusion, therefore meant that he would have to retrain to a nonconstruction job — maybe sit behind a desk and earn much less. To him, desk-sitters were "namby-pamby-types," he liked doing a man's work up on the high beams. He wanted no part of indoor work that would have him looking at the four walls and getting soft. It reminded him too much of doing school work that he never cared for very much as a kid. Sports and action and throwing and catching steel rivets were the kind of life he wanted.

One afternoon after he was coming from the office of the Georgia State vocational rehabilitation advisor, he stopped for some gasoline. At the pumps he met Dick Malloy, a high school buddy he hadn't seen for years. When asked how he had been doing, Scott uncharacteristically exclaimed, "Terrible, my ankle has ruined my whole life." He then told about the touch football injury and how it stopped him from walking the high beams.

Dick Malloy identified with the symptoms that Scott described. "I had them myself in my knee," said his friend. He then told Scott, "I've got just the physician for you. You must go and see James A. Carlson, an osteopath in Knoxville, Tennessee. He'll fix you up just the way he fixed my knee. Before getting cured, I had gone to two orthopedic specialists. Each of them sliced me open and accomplished nothing but give me pain. I wore braces and took physical therapy, and the joint still swelled and had me in agony. It gave out on me

5

constantly. Still, after Doc Carlson gave me those special reconstruction injections, I could tell right away that help was at hand. After ten months of treatments, I didn't bother with my braces; my swelling and popping disappeared, and they've never come back. That was three years ago. I even went back to playing vigorous golf and tennis that both orthopedists said I would never play again. Each one told me that my knee was just too torn up for doing anything more than take a short walk."

Scott hardly believed his friend. He said to himself, what could this osteopath in a small city like Knoxville know that the famous orthopedist in Atlanta didn't know. Besides Knoxville is about two hundred miles from Atlanta. If he drove, he might have to stay overnight and add a motel room and meals onto the cost of the doctor's visit.

But then he reasoned it out with his wife, Margie. "I've got everything I've worked for going down the drain. Don't I?"

Margie said, "Scott, the way things are going, it's miserable for both of us. I'm all for you phoning this doctor and giving his shots a try."

He made the call, but learned that it would be three months before Dr. Carlson had an open appointment on his schedule. James Carlson, D.O. of Knoxville is renowned for nonsurgical joint reconstruction, treatment that he has been administering without fanfare but with loads of success for fifteen years. The doctor's receptionist, Ann, was sympathetic but firm about giving those in need their rightful turns with the doctor, and she held out against the caller's demands.

But then Scott pleaded his case. He said that Dick Malloy told him that Dr. Carlson was his last resort. "It's the only place that can help me. Please, I've got to come in right away. My money can't hold out much longer, and I'm awfully depressed just laying around the house. My ankle won't let me work. I feel like less than a man. Please, I'll do anything the doctor wants me to do, and I can come anytime because I can't work. Please!"

Ann could tell by Scott's plaintive voice that he was sincere all right, and desperate. So, she prevailed upon Dr. Carlson to cut his lunch break to fifteen minutes in order to give the new patient some attention. Scott left Atlanta at 8:00 AM and arrived in Knoxville at noon.

After putting him through a thorough physical examination, a clinical case history, and taking diagnostic X-ray films, Dr. Carlson decided that, indeed, he could help Scott Drake by the use of reconstructive therapy, taping and gentle manipulation. Since time was vital to the patient, Dr. Carlson advised him to come for treatment once-a-week, "And don't miss a single visit until both you and I are satisfied with the result. Now I'll give you your first set of injections," he said.

The ankle swelled some more and hurt for a few days afterward, but then he noticed greater strength and stability seeming to come over the right limb. Feeling that he was finally following a good lead, Scott kept his word and made the 400 mile round-trip weekly. In two months he was able to return to work on the steel beams high above ground level, because he felt secure with a strong ankle under him. His confidence was back, depressed feelings were lifted, and money began rolling in again.

Near the end of his visits, he told Dr.Carlson, "I phoned Dick Malloy and thanked him for telling me about you and how his knee got fixed. Without the two of you, I just don't know where I'd be today. For sure, I know that I wouldn't be elevating up to the thirty-second floor of that new office building I'm working on for the next few months."

Dr. Carlson has this case history in his files. He took care of Scott Drake in the fall of 1985. Before contributing this patient story for our book, the doctor checked with his patient on August 1, 1989 and learned that the iron worker is happy at work, had no recurrence of his ankle weakness, and he and Margie have had another baby. They named their new little boy James (Jimmy), in honor of Dr. James Carlson.

Marie Philips of Beaumont, Texas is a delightful, ordinarily cheerful 74-year-old homemaker who had difficulty smiling, chewing, or even closing her jaw. She was in ongoing discomfort from temporomandibular joint (TMJ) syndrome. This chronic condition is a restriction of motion and general limitation in the hinge joint between the mandible and the temporal bones of the jaw.

In August 1985, Mrs. Philips visited John L. Sessions, D.O. of Kirbyville, Texas who examined her difficulty and treated the complaint with three nearly painless injections of sodium morrhuate, one of the many medications used for reconstructive therapy. As a result, Mrs. Philips' pain and the swelling surrounding it were completely alleviated.

Now, over four years later, the woman has maintained her correction. She told us that she can wear her dentures, chew well, smile and laugh, and care for those she cares about without any thought to the TMJ dysfunction that once had disrupted her life.

Sara Novak had been suffering with repeated migraine headaches. Her chronic pain was destroying the quality of her life. In fact, they had been with her for over thirty-nine years — ever since she was eleven years old. She accepted them as part of the burden of living, and occasionally the thought struck her — when she lingered in the throes of a migraine attack — that continuing to live was not worthwhile any longer.

One neurologist after another had tried prescription pain medicines, with no lasting relief for Mrs. Novak. In the entire City of Chicago, where she lived and worked as a bookkeeper, there was no health professional to help her. Pain-killing drugs only left the woman attempting to function while in a stupor.

Finding her way in June 1986 to the Milwaukee Pain Clinic and Metabolic Research Center, which is under the medical direction of William J. Faber, D.O., Mrs. Novak underwent laboratory and clinical examinations. She was told by Dr. Faber that the main cause of her headaches was weakened ligaments in her neck that pulled and irritated nerve endings around the spinal column. The weakness had set in four decades before from whiplash received in an automobile accident. She was sitting in the passenger's seat, then, with her father driving. While they were waiting for a red light to change, another car plowed into their rear end.

Typical whiplash injury is damage to the ligaments, vertebrae, spinal cord, and/or nerve roots in the neck region, caused by sudden jerking back of the head and neck. At its most severe, death or permanent paralysis (quadriplegia or paraplegia) may result. Sudden deceleration in a motor accident is the most common cause. Immobilization using a special collar is the principal treatment, and it is usually totally inadequate. This is what Sara Novak had undergone when she was a child. While she did not have paralysis, her migraine headaches had remained the rest of her life. Yet, suddenly, the patient found relief.

Using reconstructive therapy and some improvements in the patient's diet, Dr. Faber relieved Mrs. Novak of her migraines in nine weekly sessions. Speaking of her experience, the patient said, "It was like getting my life back again after going through almost forty years of hell."

A long-time sufferer of pain in both hands and in the right knee, a hardware salesman from Canfield, Ohio, Richard Desh, age 59, visited holistic physician L. Terry Chappell, M.D. Dr. Chappell is medical director of the Celebration of

Health Center of Bluffton, Ohio and former President of the Great Lakes Association of Clinical Medicine. Mr. Desh had heard from others that this physician was using an advanced technique with remarkable success for the elimination of chronic joint pain. A retired music professor had mentioned to him about good results he had received from joint reconstruction of his knees. Then Mr. Desh heard of the treatment again from his sister-in-law who told of her neighbor who had her stiff and inflamed bunion (called hallux valgus) treated with this new injection technique and was able to avoid surgery.

Now, Canfield is approximately 170 miles, east of Bluffton, but the patient decided to make the trip anyway. Hearing good things about one small town doctor and the treatment he is administering in another small town over such a long distance is not to be denied. It was worth a try, Mr. Desh told us.

From the history obtained by Dr. Chappell's nurse, it was evident that Richard Desh had a tendency toward unstable joints. He had experienced trauma with tearing of the medial collateral ligament in his right knee ten years before. A nerve had been rerouted in his left elbow due to its being compressed from chronic inflammation, and a herniated lumbar disc had been removed by an orthopedic surgeon from his lower back two years before.

The elbow and back did not bring him to Dr. Chappell. And although he limped slightly from discomfort in his knee, the man's major problem was both of his hands. His thumbs were swollen. They were almost immobile from weakness and stiffness. The muscles at the base of both thumbs were enlarged almost twice the normal size. In his work at the hardware store, Mr. Desh found that he could not pick up dollar bills from the register to make change. If he dropped a nail while counting out the number being purchased, he was unable to pick it up from the floor. Turning pages of a telephone book was difficult. Attempting to turn pages in church was actually unpleasant — the process for him being so slow and tedious — that the scripture was read completely before he could find the appropriate page to follow along. Shaking anybody's hand was excruciating, and he avoided it. He felt self-conscious about being considered unfriendly.

The patient tried one arthritic medication after another. He came to the conclusion that television commercials simply lie. For instance, he had recently tried Feldene™, but it only led to his experiencing burning gastritis and the necessity to buffer it with Tagamet™.

Checking his joints by X-ray, Dr. Chappell saw that Mr. Desh had only slight calcium spurring on the edge of the patella (kneecap), but the carpometacarpal joints (where the thumbs begin) showed that the joint spaces were narrowing and spur formation and "sclerosis" or thickening of the articulating surfaces were present.

Dr. Chappell took the patient off all medication and started him on a multivitamin program to build up his stamina and immunity. His biochemistry was checked and found to be adequate. Digestion was good and the man had two bowel movements daily. Being metabolically normal in bowel habits and digestion is quite important for assurance of success with joint reconstruction.

Nonsurgical reconstructive therapy was begun for Mr. Desh. His knee proved to be more of an inflammatory problem than a chronic structural one, and a single session of knee injections completely eliminated his pain. No further treatment was need then, or after.

The patient's impaired thumbs followed a more typical pattern of response to therapy. Mr. Desh felt discomfort from the first set of injections the same evening. He had swelling, but then he experienced three days of solid relief. He was able to work more effectively in the hardware store during this period than in the previous ten years.

The first few sessions resulted in his dramatic improvement in function. He traveled the 340 miles roundtrip once a week. Initially Richard Desh noticed a few more aches and pains in other areas due to the withdrawal he was experiencing from the Feldene™, but this slight discomfort went away over time. Gradually, swelling of his thumbs went away, and the man's ability to make careful coordinated movements with his hands improved. However, after the fourth injection treatment (not with sodium morrhuate, since it is contraindicated for use in the small joints of the hands and feet), he noticed some added tenderness in the skin where the needle punctures had been made. Subsequently, Dr. Chappell added ethyl chloride coolant spray as a numbing agent for the skin prior to the injections. Relief was immediate.

Fine movements of his hands were restored to Mr. Desh once again. He required six series of injections to make his hand ligaments strong enough for his joint symptoms to be corrected. At the completion of his reconstructive therapy he could easily count out nuts and bolts and make change. Worship on Sunday became pleasurable for him once again. He could follow the scripture along with everyone else. And at the end of the last treatment visit, Richard Desh gave Dr. L. Terry Chappell a good firm handshake with a big smile instead of a grimace of pain.

Chapter Two
What Is Reconstructive Therapy?

A retired naval officer and past president of the Pennnsylvania Blue Shield health insurance corporation — the patient of Harold C. Walmer, D.O., F.A.O.A.S., D.M.A., of Elizabethtown, Pennsylvania — is anxious to help us describe what is reconstructive therapy. He wishes others to know of benefits one may receive from this treatment for chronic joint, tendon, and ligament pain. Consequently, he wrote a letter to us, signing his name and his address, and giving us permission to use both. We have decided to publish his letter without altering it, except for changing his reference word, "sclerotherapy," to "reconstructive therapy." Moreover, in conformity with the rule laid down by the individual state medical societies against using patients' true identities, we have given him a pseudonym — Ralph Everett Ralston of Harrison, Pennsylvania. Mr. Ralston writes the following to us:

Reconstructive therapy? Never heard of it! But when I did and investigated further, I learned that the procedure was considered experimental — and yes, even controversial — in some medical quarters and among some of your own osteopathic colleagues. However, if one is in severe pain, does not like gulping twelve or fourteen aspirins a day to alleviate it, and does not relish the prospect of prolonged traction or surgical tinkering as a remedy, then he or she is certainly not averse to the consideration of reconstructive therapy.

Such was my case when in the winter of 1977 I was suddenly struck by sciatica and acute pain in the lower back. I could not stand up in an erect position; had great difficulty sitting; and worst of all — intermittent sleep was the rule of the night. Rather depressed, I wondered if ever there was to be light at the end of the tunnel. Then by chance a friend told me about Harold Walmer, D.O. of Elizabethtown, Pennsylvania.

I first visited Dr. Walmer in April, 1977. In discussing my sorry state of affairs, I did manage to ask if I ever would play golf again. His response was most gratifying. In explaining his philosophy of the conservative treatment of lower back pain by reconstructive therapy, Dr. Walmer said that he could not promise one the moon, but that he felt confident the procedure would help correct my problems. And further — my eyes must have lit up when he said that I would be able to swing a golf club again — and perhaps even better! I was 61 years of age at the time.

Apparently age had begun to take its toll. The diagnosis was an inflammation of the sciatic nerve and osteoarthritis. To me it was still a "helluva" lot of pain. One of the contributing factors which Dr. Walmer discovered and which was not detected by any doctor during my civilian and naval careers up to that time was that my right leg was shorter than the left, causing pelvic imbalance. So, the first step in treatment was to put a 3/16" lift in the right heel of all my shoes. Then ensued treatments through reconstructive therapy, totaling 12 in number. As I recall the first treatments were about twice a week and later treatments were spaced out over a longer period of time as my condition improved and, in turn, my spirits began to rise again.

Within a couple of months I was as happy as I could be whacking that ball on the links! But what is more remarkable is that I was able to remain mobile while I

14

was undergoing treatment. I did not miss a day of work [at Pennsylvania Blue Shield]. Moreover, the total cost of the sessions of reconstructive therapy was certainly less than that which would have been incurred if surgery had been performed on an in-patient basis in the hospital.

Just as back surgery may not be the remedy for everyone, reconstructive therapy may not be the "remedy ticket" for everyone who has severe lower back pain. Still, the simple fact remains that the conservative route of reconstructive therapy before any surgery did work for me. And it has proved to be effective even nine years later.

In 1986 I encountered sciatica again since the aging process never stops. Consequently, I had further reconstructive therapy which remedied the problem. Today, March 6, 1989, at the age of 73 I am looking forward to playing golf tomorrow.

Defining Reconstructive Therapy

Nonsurgical reconstructive therapy (also still referred to by some health professionals as prolotherapy, sclerotherapy or proliferative therapy) is the introduction of an irritant solution by means of injection into weakened areas of the body. The irritant brings about proliferation of tissue, making the involved areas permanently stronger. The tissue proliferation, as previously emphasized, provides the main side effect of reconstructive therapy — more joint endurance and less chronic pain. The injected solution mostly goes into the damaged ligaments, tendons, and surrounding joint capsules.

The ligaments are the supporting structures — fibrous bands (like strong rubber bands) — connecting bones that come together (articulating bones). Bones articulate or move when they join at a point where their opposing surfaces are lined with lubricating tissue that prevents friction and grinding. Examples are cartilaginous, fibrous, or soft (synovial) tissues. The function of ligaments is to hold joints together. If the ligaments are too loose from injury, repeated motion, wear and tear, or degenerative arthritis, the individual develops a loose joint that does not function properly. It continues to slip and slide out of the track it was designed to follow.

Ligaments are to be distinguished from tendons (which are attached to muscle). Tendons lie over a joint and are one tissue layer above the bone and ligaments. The tendons and muscles move the joints, but the ligaments hold the joints together and limit the range of motion of a joint. At one of its ends, a tendon is attached to a muscle and to a bone of a joint at the other. Ligaments attach one bone of a joint to another bone of that same joint.

Generally torn or stretched ligaments and tendons do not heal on their own because tendons and ligaments don't enjoy the influx of good blood supply present in other areas. Therefore, the goal of reconstructive therapy is to produce sufficient controlled irritation within the ligament, tendon, or joint being treated so as to stimulate your body to create tissue that strengthens the weak body part. Such stimulation produces a more durable fibrous band. The body responds to irritation from the proliferant (the irritating solution) by laying down extra ligament-like tissue. Thus, a controlled biochemical reaction is created by the doctor who administers the injection. It occurs within or around your joint. By introduction of the irritant via reconstructive therapy, a slight inflammation is built up. This signals the body to increase the blood supply to the injected area. The result is that fibroblasts (healing cells) travel to this irritated spot and lay down repair tissue within and around it.

From employing reconstructive therapy, eventually — usually sooner rather than later — chronic joint pain goes away — and stays away permanently. The benefits from this procedure start almost immediately when the injections are given by a well-trained nonsurgical joint reconstruction therapist. As the patient, you will feel increased joint, ligament, and tendon stability, greater strength, and more endurance.

At the fibro-osseous junction — the place where ligaments originate and attach to the bones that comprise a joint — the injected solution causes the production of fibrous tissue precursor cells, or "proles." You then have the creation, through a process of rapid, profuse buildup of proles, of an internal 'weld' stabilizing the joint. A success rate of about 88 percent is reported by the approximately 250 physicians in the United States and Canada who routinely utilize this technique. Those patients who don't gain benefits generally have various metabolic difficulties in their bodies which interfere with ordinary healing of poorly nourished internal tissues. (Good healing of the skin does not count as a predictor of reconstructive treatment success, since, unlike ligaments and tendons, the skin is an external tissue with fine nourishment from an excellent blood supply.)

Reasons Why the Procedure Is Still Finding Its Name

A well-experienced reconstruction therapist, Kent Pomeroy, M.D., of Phoenix, Arizona, who participated in a round table discussion about the procedure during mid-1985 at the American Association of Orthopedic Medicine, stated: "The names [prolotherapy and sclerotherapy] are misleading. Prolotherapy was the name coined by Hackett [George Stuart Hackett, M.D., F.A.C.S., consulting surgeon at Mercy Hospital of Canton, Ohio, of whom we will have more to say later] a number of years ago. The purpose of his coining this word was to indicate that there is a fibrous regeneration or proliferation of tissue [the prolos] produced by injected sub-

17

stances. Sclerotherapy is not a completely accurate term either as it applies to ligaments and tendons. 'Sclero' implies that only scar tissue has been regenerated while research with laboratory animals revealed that actual ligamentous and tendinous prototype tissues are regenerated and not just scar tissue.

"The general public has a mistaken view whenever we use these terms. In fact, the medical and osteopathic societies, themselves, generally have a misunderstanding of what these terms mean because of the terms themselves. A number of terms that are more accurate could replace 'prolo' or 'sclero.' There is a regeneration or a genesis of fibrous tissue (ligamentous and tendinous) at the fibrosseous junction with the bone."

Another round table participant, James Carlson, D.O., of Knoxville, Tennessee, replied, " 'Nonsurgical joint reconstruction' is the term that should be used, particularly on the spinal ligaments, those that are not amenable to surgical access or to surgical reconstruction. This includes the ligaments of the pelvis. It does not have to be restricted to those joints, however."

The more descriptive term, once preferred by co-author William J. Faber, D.O., 'proliferative therapy,' has an obvious derivation. It indicates the technique of injecting solutions into tissue for the purpose of proliferation of prolos, the new fibrous tissue.

Writing in the American Journal of Acupuncture, Louis Vanderschot, D.O. of Dallas, Texas calls reconstructive therapy "the American version of acupuncture."[1] Dr. Vanderschot points out that one of the many modern applications of acupuncture is aquapuncture (the hypodermic injection of water to produce counterirritation or for any other purpose), and aquapuncture has a history of being practiced in the United States as far back as the early 1950s in the form

18

of reconstructive therapy.

The History of Reconstructive Therapy

In various forms, reconstructive therapy has been available and used in medicine for thousands of years. In the Fifth Century, B.C., Hippocrates treated separated shoulders of wounded soldiers with cauterizing irons. His crude technique was highly successful and continued to be applied for a long period in medical history. Cauterization causes the body to lay down fibrous tissue in response to the irritation of burning. While effective and not at all like today's joint reconstruction, Hippocrates' method was hard on the patient. He made it clear that he had the proper approach to the problem when he described his technique.

Hippocrates began by saying: "It deserves to be known how a shoulder which is subject to frequent dislocations should be treated. I have never known any physician to treat the case properly, and some physicians abandon the attempt altogether while others practice the very reverse of what is proper." These physicians being criticized by Hippocrates, some 2,500 years ago, were cauterizing at the top of the shoulder. Hippocrates went on to explain the proper procedure. He said to raise the patient's arm about halfway up and make a couple of quick vertical cuts in the armpit with a red-hot cautery. "The cauteries should be red-hot," he cautioned, "so that they may pass through as quickly as possible." The resultant scars would provide the necessary support to keep the shoulder from dislocating, Hippocrates declared, and he was proven correct over the next few millennia. [2]

About 145 years ago, a French physician named Alfred A. L. M. Velpeau (also spelled Valpeau), the doctor who gave medicine the Velpeau bandage (the sling), injected an iodine solution of carbolic acid (phenol) to produce scar tissue. This strengthened the abdominal muscles of his patients. His

19

method was meant for the treatment of hernias, and it worked.[3]

About fifty-five years ago (since the advent of the modern syringe) the entire procedure began to become refined. In 1935, Abram Lippman, M.D. successfully used the injection of sclerosing solutions for the correction without surgery of inguinal hernias. The usefulness of reconstructive therapy (then called sclerotherapy) was enhanced as techniques were further developed in 1936 for hemorrhoids, for varicose veins, and for esophageal varices in alcoholism. Earl Gedney, D.O. extended the uses of sclerosing solutions, in 1937, to correct weakened knee and low back joints. He applied a solution manufactured by G.D. Searle called Sylnasol, the sodium salt of the unsaturated fatty acids of linseed oil.[4] Seeing Dr. Gedney's excellent results, other physicians utilized similar techniques for temporomandibular joint (TMJ) problems, cervical spine and head injuries, and again for varicose veins and inguinal hernias.

In the same year, Louis Schultz, M.D., was using the same solution to treat weak TMJ problems, as well, but he utilized a technique that differed from Dr. Gedney's.[5] David Shuman, D.O., who performed early work on joint reconstruction with the Late Earl Gedney at the Philadelphia College of Osteopathic Medicine, told of these experiences in *Osteopathic Annals.*[6] He wrote, "Dr. Schultz' technique differed from ours in that he injected the solution into the joint, whereas all those I know who treat weak joints inject into the ligaments. After 1937 more techniques evolved, and in 1941 I published a paper, *Luxation Recurring in Shoulder,*[7] and I kept in mind what Hippocrates said about going into the armpit. . . . Dr. Gedney went to Bangor, Maine, and became chief surgeon at the Bangor Osteopathic Hospital. While there, he developed a technique for injecting the lateral reflection of the anterior spinal ligament that proved to be very helpful in cases of herniated disk. He published his results in an article titled *Disk Syndrome*."[8]

Dr. Schuman explained that the American Osteopathic Academy of Sclerotherapy came into being somewhat after that. "Sylnasol is no longer made," he wrote, "however, a solution very similar to it, sodium morrhuate, the unsaturated fatty acids of cod liver oil, is used by me and many others. There are a number of solutions being used according to the individual physician's preference." In fact, literally dozens of medications — drugs and nutrients, alike — are administered as proliferating agents for purposes of stimulating the formation of new fibrous tissue. When the prolos are laid down, the supporting ligament becomes thicker, firmer, and seemingly more adherent to the bone at its attachments.

Dr. George Stuart Hackett

In 1956, a general surgeon who performed orthopedic surgery, George Stuart Hackett, M.D., F.A.C.S., published a little known monograph purporting to show that many chronic low back problems were the result of stretching or tearing of ligaments around the joints of the spine and pelvis.[9] He injected a proliferating agent directly into the bone-attachment sites of torn vertebral ligaments. It was Dr. Hackett's contention that in many individuals the normal healing process following injuries or strains was inadequate, resulting in a weakness of the attachment of the ligament to bone.

As it happens, Dr. Hackett's small book was not at all insignificant. *Ligament and Tendon Relaxation (Skeletal Disability) Treated by Prolotherapy (Fibro-Osseous Proliferation)* formed the basis for a major breakthrough in the treatment of chronic joint pain. It's an advancement in the correction of human misery that stands on a par with the discovery of penicillin, the artificial production of insulin, or Joseph Lister's concepts of sterile technique for surgery. In the monograph's preface to the third edition, Dr. Hackett described his work: ". . . for the first time in history the most frequent cause of chronic painful skeletal disability has been definitely established. A method of confirming the diagnosis and a successful treatment have been developed. Within the attachment of weakened ligaments and tendons to bone, the sensory nerves become overstimulated by abnormal tension to become not only the origin of specific local pain, but also definite areas of referred pain throughout the body to as far as the head, fingers and toes from specific relaxed ligaments and tendons."

It is commonly stated by those trained in reconstructive therapy that Dr. Hackett later in his career reported his treatment successful for 1,600 patients over a 19-year period. Remarkably, 82 percent of Hackett's patients were found to be cured of backache during the followup examinations administered by outside observing clinicians. (The current success rate has now been increased to 88 percent by improved injection procedures and the use of solutions that are less apt to bring on allergic reactions in the patients.) These 1600 patients of Hackett's were people who had each undergone a series of injections for chronic joint pain. Their pain had been present, it is said, for variable periods. But the relief they experienced after treatment was completed ranged from a minimum of two years duration to a maximum of twelve years. The injection benefits had remained for them during that entire period. Of those examined, 253 patients had suffered with sacroiliac joint weakness, a most difficult back problem to cure. Still later, Dr. Hackett reported successful results in the treatment of spondylolisthesis, a condition in which the back vertebrae slip forward or backward on each other as a result of ligamentous weakness. Because of his publication of clinical results in medical journals, ongoing research, and the teaching of his methods to other physicians, George S. Hackett is considered the true grandfather of modern joint reconstructive therapy.

In 1961 Dr. Hackett and three colleagues, T.C. Huang, Ph.D., Alan Raftery, M.D., and Theodore J. Dodd, M.D, reported even more dramatic results in the journal *Military Medicine*. In an eight year experiment, over variable periods ranging up to one year, the achilles tendons of 192 live New Zealand white rabbits were checked to determine the amount of new bone and fibrous tissue that was induced following injections of proliferative materials. In this same article, he reported on 21 years of management of 1,857 patients with ligament relaxation. They ranged in ages from 15 to 88 and had suffered from the disability from three months to 65 years. In the most significant finding yet, 82 percent of the patients were cured.[10]

Even among those practicing the discipline of reconstructive therapy, not many know that Dr. Hackett published a second book in 1968, *Myoneurovascular Mechanisms. Disease Prevention. Prolotherapy*[11]. In it he summarized nearly everything that he had uncovered in his perfection of the osteopathic/orthopedic discipline that has come to be known as nonsurgical joint reconstructive therapy.

Today, reconstructive therapy is applied with better results, although with less publicity, than most types of back surgery. For example, according to the *Journal of Bone and Joint Surgery*, surgical intervention for disk involvement (unstable lower back syndrome) is satisfactory in only approximately half of the people operated on. In comparison, as we have stated, during Dr. Hackett's experimental period of treatment about 35 years ago, 82 percent of reconstructive therapy recipients had success, while over 88 percent of patients receiving the injection procedure today experience permanent correction. They no longer are victims of unstable lower back syndromes. The current statistical rate of cure for all types of chronic joint pain injected with proliferants is reaching toward 92 percent.

Chapter Three

Chronic Joint Pain and Your Ligaments

"I am a well-experienced professional dancer and earn my living by offering instruction in the dance to children in and around Sheboygen, Wisconsin.

"Actually I've been confronting three musculoskeletal problems with which I must cope. Any one of them could end my dancing career quite suddenly. A congenitally short first metatarsal in my right foot — a condition called Morton's syndrome — is causing me imbalance and deformity with the onset of a bunion. I have a chronically weak left ankle arising from pulled ligaments which came from two severe sprains that struck four and five years ago. Finally, the worst of my three disabilities, scollosis, produces back spasms that strike me periodically. The spasms created loss of movement and reduce range of motion for me. Any one of these musculoskeletal problems offer an uncertain future for someone who depends on her dancing ability as a teaching instrument."

For purpose of definition, scollosis is a lateral curvature of the spine, named according to the location and direction of the convexity, most often in the thoracic region. You see, the spinal column, composed of thirty-three vertebrae — connected blocks — is shaped somewhat like the letter **S** if seen from the side. The portion in the neck and loin region are curved convex forward; in the thoracic and lowest region concave forward. The spine has springiness and elasticity which protect the brain and other organs from constant shocks and jolts. In scollosis there usually are two curves, the original and a compensatory curve — for example, an original right thoracic with a compensatory left curve in the loin region.

"I had contacted many doctors. They all suggested some form of surgery as correction, but none of them offered any guarantee that the operation would bring me back to good repair. The other option was for me to learn to live with the condition."

The Situation Takes a Turn for the Better

"My mother attended a workshop of the Wisconsin Natural Health Association, and she brought me some literature that described reconstructive therapy at the Milwaukee Pain Clinic. After consulting Dr. Faber at the clinic, he decided to start me on recontructive therapy, first with injections into my ankle. Yes, the needling is uncomfortable, but the gradual strengthening of my ankle made the temporary discomfort all worthwhile.

"I now have a better range of motion, more flexibility, plus firm tissue structures around the ankle joint. I've not had to tape the damaged area in over two years because now the ligaments are firm and strong enough to sustain themselves.

"The doctor has been doing the same thing for my right foot and back. My previously dysfunctional areas are becoming as strong now in my middle years as when I was a young girl."

The Vital Role Ligaments Play in Joint Stability

What do you know about the ligaments and tendons of your body and the vital role they play in holding together your skeleton? If you answer, "Not very much!" you'll be joining crowds of others, including some doctors. Few persons really understand that primarily ligaments and to a lesser degree, tendons, hold the joints in place. The muscles do not.

The ligament surrounding a joint is a band of flexible,

tough, dense white fibrous connective tissue. It is so closely attached to each joint that if the joint is put under great stress or strain as in an automobile accident, a severe fall, or from lifting a heavy object, the ligament must stretch or be torn. If overstretched constantly, it eventually tears or becomes a chronically loose joint binder. Then, articulating bones will fall out of place and joint dislocation (subluxation) occurs. The result? Pain strikes suddenly or slowly. Sudden pain might feel like a stabbing knife. Slow pain could become a steadily building ache and sense of pressure. The speed and intensity of resulting pain depend on the extent of joint subluxation.

What causes the pain? Sensory nerves carry messages to the brain that all is not well. Sensory nerves within the ligaments are convoluted, looping back within their fibrous bands. When the bands are stressed, the nerves get put under tension causing aching and pulling warnings to be sent to the brain. Problems could arise at any site on the skeleton where bones join with other bones to form an articulation (a joint, the junction of two or more bones).

Nerves come away from the spine in different areas to either supply your internal organs or affect them by reflex. Spinal dislocations or subluxations will eventually lower the resistance to a given internal organ. The organ is affected by the nerve supplying it which arises from around this subluxated spinal joint. A spinal subluxation as, for instance, the subluxation of the first rib on the left side, can be the direct cause of tachycardia (too fast a heart rate). Furthermore, a subluxation at the fourth dorsal vertebra can also affect the function of the heart. Spinal nerves arising from different subluxations may adversely affect the gall bladder, stomach, appendix, colon, small intestine, and other organs. Many internal problems can develop from lax ligaments not holding the spinal articulations in proper alignment. That singular concept forms the basis for the entire therapeutic program of the chiropractic profession.

The cause of pain for you could be quite distant from the pain itself. For that reason, pain in the toes, foot, ankle, or knee may be coming from a subluxation of the spine at the sacroiliac. Until correction of this spinal subluxation is achieved, you might spend much time, money, and suffering for some other unnecessarily sophisticated treatment that fails to work. Yet, your condition could very well be more simply corrected by reconstructive therapy or another osteopathic technique such as manipulation. To accomplish success in treatment, the trick is to have a proper diagnosis. Thus to discover the reason for chronic joint pain being present, uncovering the sites of dysfunctional ligaments and/or tendons is the key to diagnosis and eventual cure with reconstructive therapy.

Structural relationships in the skeleton depend to a great extent upon the ligaments that hold joints in proper position. These supporting thongs hold the bones and joints in place and also support the organs. They do not stretch but are interlaced so as to permit movements. The ligaments connecting the vertebrae are more elastic and allow a considerable range of motion, as in bending the back.

Chronic Joint Pain Transmission and Response

In its many forms, ranging from sharp stabs to dull aches, pain demands attention. The word pain derives from the Greek term for penalty, suggesting an ancient perception that pain is a price we pay for living.

Although acute pain can be excruciating, it's usually both transient and purposeful. But when pain becomes chronic, it loses meaning and threatens well-being. As differentiated from acute pain which is highly localized, usually sharp, occasionally radiating, and generally arising from an acute injury or disease, chronic joint pain is poorly localized, dull, constant, and nagging. It may be intractable and have an ill-defined source.

In the prior section on ligament involvement with unstable joints, illustrated by subluxation of the vertebrae, we referred to nerves as a first stop on the pain pathway. The peripheral nervous system (PNS), which includes spinal sensory nerves and dorsal root ganglion cells in the spinal cord, provides a communications network for the central nervous system (CNS). Working together, the PNS and the CNS receive, transmit, and interpret sensory pain messages and regulate the body's responses to them.

Pain impulses are regulated by substances that act at various points along the pain pathways. Prostaglandins, potent fatty acids that stimulate a wide range of effects, are synthesized within cells after cell membrane injury, as occurs in joint instability. Other chemical regulators called endorphins are opiate-like substances called opioid peptides that modulate pain through several different mechanisms. They bind with opiate receptor sites throughout the nervous system and inhibit release of such neurotransmitters as something referred to by scientists as substance "P." Pain perception is altered. Aspirin, for instance, has a substance P that stimulates the formation of endorphins.

There are three major, traditional theories to explain the basic concepts of pain reception:

The **gate control** theory states that pain is modulated by a mechanism in the spinal cord and higher CNS structures which open and close neurological sensitivities.

The **pattern theory** says that pain impulses generated by receptors form a pattern or code, that informs the CNS that pain is present.

The oldest theory of pain, the **specificity theory**, assumes that pain travels from specific pain receptors to a pain center in the brain and that the relationship between a stimulus and response is direct, uniform, and invariable.

In addition there is a fourth pair of concepts that are widely accepted by those adapting Dr. Hackett's methods of reconstructive therapy.

The Hackett Concepts of Trigger Point Pain and Referred Pain

In his monograph on ligament and tendon relaxation, Dr. Hackett expounds on two related new-but-old concepts: **trigger point pain** and referred pain.[1] He focused on chronic joint pain, in particular. His concept was that "sensory impulses arise chiefly in the ligaments, which crisscross and run in various directions to maintain stability of the articulations in all positions. We are not aware of these impulses during our ordinary activities, for they merely help us keep upright and aid the body in its movements. When a normal ligament is submitted to excessive traction or strain at its fibro-periosteal junction [the spot where ligament attaches to bone]," continued Dr. Hackett, "the sensory impulse is of such intensity that it reaches consciousness and a release of traction is voluntarily accomplished.

"When the fibrous strands of the ligament become relaxed or weakened from any cause [as with the ankle sprain of Michael Resk], a normal tension on the ligament causes a stretching or elongation of the fibrous stands of the ligament, and this elongation permits an abnormal tension-stimulation of the intraligamentous nerve fibrils which will not stretch. This is the cause of the local or trigger point pain in ligament relaxation," Dr. Hackett concluded.

Trigger point pain may be described by the victim as feeling dull, aching, sharp, piercing, burning, boring, drilling, shooting, numb, dead feeling, itching, pricking, squeezing, compression, pressure, tired, heavy, or pulling. "A brief weak stimulation usually results in local pain only, but when the stimulation is prolonged and/or intense, there is often an accompanying referred pain," he added.

Trigger point pain is important to the diagnostician, wrote Dr. Hackett, because (1) it is useful to locate the exact ligament or tendon that is damaged, (2) it confirms the diagnosis by its being needled, and (3) it helps the doctor place his needle to deliver an injection of proliferant solution.

President John F. Kennedy's personal physician, Janet Travell, M.D., was famous for her interligamentous use of local anesthetic to eliminate trigger point pain. Dr. Travell reported that pain in sacroiliac disability may be referred throughout the sciatic distribution into the buttock, outer thigh and leg to just above the inner ankle. She wrote, "Referred pain induced from injection or needling of trigger points persists for several minutes and its distribution can usually be clearly delineated by the subject."

In a 1954 medical journal article, Dr. Hackett points out that he has reproduced local and referred pains by the same type of irritation with the needle described by Dr. Travell and by pressure of a local anesthetic delivered into the area by syringe. The pains disappear entirely within two minutes as the action of the anesthetic takes place, he said.[2] This is a method similar to neural therapy developed by two West Germans, the brothers Ferdinand Huneke, M.D. and Walter Huneke, M.D.[3]

In an unpublished paper, Kent L. Pomeroy, M.D. of Phoenix, Arizona did an historical review of Dr. Hackett's combination theory of trigger point pain and referred pain. "Basically," Dr. Pomeroy writes, "Hackett contends that once a ligament or tendon becomes incompetent due to strain, sprain, or tearing, and if it remains incompetent because of inadequate healing, then pain may be associated with these same tissues by stretching of the fibers under normal tension. This happens because there is now a conflict between the relaxed ligament or tendon which will stretch, and the non-elastic sensory nerves within the ligament or tendon, which do not normally stretch. The result is an abnormal stimulation of the sensory nerves and this is interpreted at the conscious level as pain."

In his own November, 1956 published article, Dr. Hackett wrote a description of the source of referred pain, using medical language. He said:[4]

> When the ligament fibers become relaxed, a normal tension will then produce a bombardment of afferent somatic proprioceptive sensory impulses from the ligament into the spinal posterior root ganglion [nerves receiving messages from the rest of the body into the spinal cord], where some are transmitted to the brain as consciousness of local pain, while other impulses in some way stimulate exteroceptive impulses which also enter consciousness as superficial pain from an area which has its sensory distribution from the same spinal segment and is known as the referred pain area.

The source of pain located in any part of the body, but especially in the case of back pain and referred pain in the lower limbs, is therefore designated by Dr. Hackett as originating in tendons and ligaments surrounding joints where they attach into bones. He drew detailed diagrammatic maps of pain on the surface of the body. The skin maps show exact locations of referred pain that stem from trigger pain points (see Figures 1 and 2).

Finally, Dr. Hackett, in 1961, published his concept of a vicious cycle of ligament relaxation and bone decalcification in which either may induce the other. Osteoporosis, for instance, may be stimulated to occur from "loose joints" arising from ligament laxity. There will be a weakening of the fibro-osseous junction and pain at that junction. Reconstructive therapy is the means to building new bone tissue.[5]

HEAD-NECK DISABILITY

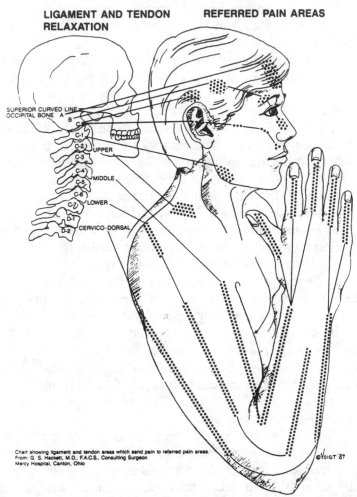

LIGAMENT AND TENDON RELAXATION

REFERRED PAIN AREAS

SUPERIOR CURVED LINE
OCCIPITAL BONE   A   B

C-1
C-2
C-3   UPPER
C-4
C-5   MIDDLE
C-6
C-7   LOWER
D-1
D-2   CERVICO-DORSAL

Chart showing ligament and tendon areas which send pain to referred pain areas.
From: G. S. Hackett, M.D., F.A.C.S., Consulting Surgeon
Mercy Hospital, Canton, Ohio

©VOIGT '87

Figure 1. Referred pain areas described by George S. Hackett, M.D. from ligaments damaged in the cervical spine. Pain is felt in the hand, arm, shoulder, face, and head.

32

LOW BACK DISABILITY

REFERRED PAIN AREAS

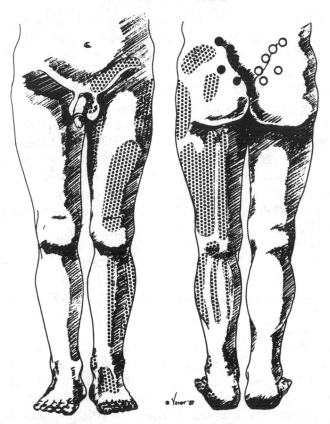

AREAS OF LOW BACK AND LEG PAIN FROM UNSTABLE LOW BACK LIGAMENTS.

● LARGE CIRCLES SHOW INVOLVED UNSTABLE LIGAMENTS.
· SMALL CIRCLES SHOW PAIN AREAS REFERRED FROM INVOLVED UNSTABLE LIGAMENTS.

Chart showing ligament and tendon areas which send pain to referred pain areas.
From: G. S. Hackett, M.D., F.A.C.S., Consulting Surgeon
Mercy Hospital, Canton, Ohio

Figure 2. From the damaged low back, referred areas of pain to the buttock, the groin, the testicles or vulvar, the leg, and the foot which were described by George S. Hackett, M.D.

Two rheumatologists, in 1971, R.G. Howes, M.D. and I.C. Isdale, M.D., validated Dr. Hackett's concepts of loose joints when they wrote on "the loose body" syndrome. They said:[6]

> Among those patients in whom an anatomical diagnosis could not be reached were a large number of women and a much smaller number of men. When the clinical findings of these cases were analyzed a pattern emerged; these patients had the onset of backache early, usually in their teens, their backache was recurrent and invariably localized to the lower lumbar area, there was a marked lumbar lordosis, and there were localized areas of diminished movements with pain at the extremes of movement, but excessive mobility of other joints . . . A major group of this survey of backache cases exhibit both spinal and peripheral ligamentous laxity . . .

So it is that Dr. George Hackett laid the groundwork with his fourth theory of pain production and pain reception — the combination of ligamentous pain trigger points and ligamentous pain referrals, with their detailed body maps of pain location.

For skilled clinicians — the proponents and users of joint reconstruction —Dr. Hackett has produced a case for what they are convinced is a valuable therapeutic tool. They administer it because of their belief that the treatment has high likelihood of success and a low risk of adverse side effects. The opponents of this technique, in contrast, consider it neither sound nor without potential for unfavorable reactions. Yet nearly all of the time these opponents of joint reconstruction have never received the treatment, nor have they administered it to others. In fact, opponents of reconstructive therapy are only conjecturing in their condemnations. They have no idea of how the treatment works within the tissues to permanently eliminate chronic joint pain.

Chapter Four

Freedom from Pain by Building New Joints, Ligaments, and Tendons

People who suffer with chronic joint pain have likely heard from their physicians simple words similar to the following: "You're just going to have to live with it. You need to accept the pain as a permanent part of your life."

These can be outrageous words — devastating, shocking, unjust, and disappointing in the extreme. The doctor says them usually when finally he or she has run out of things to do for you. Pain pills, hot packs, physical therapy, acupuncture, hypnosis, biofeedback, self-analysis, relaxation imagery, cortisone shots, nerve blocks, TENS units, surgery, or other techniques have failed to bring prolonged relief. The doctor has come to the end of the line in finding a means of restoring a wholeness to your life.

Chronic joint pain, indeed, appears to be the ultimate in cruel experience brought on by everyday living. It results in confusion, frustration, anger, loss of job, financial ruin, destroyed self-esteem, destruction of function, depression, terror, and sometimes genuine mental breakdown. Reflexes from unending joint pain trigger far-reaching responses, with ever more effects on your life. The pain behavior itself becomes controlling. It dominates the character, quality, and entire structure of your existence. It becomes so habitual that you may forget that having pain is abnormal. You don't remember what normal waking and sleeping moments are like, because you become so used to suffering and general discomfort.

Anxiety, discouragement, hopelessness, misery — your entire persona as projected — are the most common emotions you feel and show to others.

In 1956, Pope Pius XII explained to a group of visiting cardiovascular surgeons:

> Bodily pain affects man as a whole down to the deepest layers of his moral being. It forces him to face again the fundamental questions of his fate, of his attitude toward God and fellow man, of his individual and collective responsibility and of the sense of his pilgrimage on earth.

The Profile of Chronic Joint Pain

The profile of chronic joint pain — a highly penetrating and unpleasant sensation — is indicative of a physiological disorder at the attachments with bone of ligaments, tendons, cartilage, disk, and/or arthritic deposits. As described by Dr. Hackett, it is produced by irritation of the trunk, root, or terminal of a sensory nerve. Joint pain may be considered a protective mechanism in that it directs attention to some disturbance in a bony articulation. It varies with the cause and site and among different people, some persons being more sensitive to it than others.

From two viewpoints physiological and psychological an unstable joint brings on pain sensation by highly intricate mechanisms. It brings on sensations that may be described as aching, boring, gnawing, cutting, burning, or throbbing. The description of the type of pain often helps to illuminate its cause.

Although gate control and other pain theories mentioned in the last chapter do attempt to explain the physiological complexities of joint pain, all fall short of fully defining the pain phenomenon. No pain, from the slightest tinge to the most severe ache, is purely organic. Rather, every pain is a combination of a physical sensation and an emotional response.

Each individual's personality influences how he or she reacts to pain. There are four types of sufferers: (1) the augmenter who amplifies pain sensation by focusing on it, (2) the minimizer who ignores or represses it, (3) the introvert, who won't talk about it, and (4) the neurotic, who is anxious, emotionally labile, and highly sensitive to pain. Also, joint pain can be a psychiatric symptom which is easily misdiagnosed by the health care professional who doesn't have training in reconstructive therapy.

Some reconstruction therapists have developed questionnaires for patients to assess sociocultural influences which could be affecting his or her pain. Other doctors have created questionnaires for evaluating chronic joint pain in particular parts of the body which relate to actual physical encumbrances brought on by the pain. For example, in 1987, four physicians collaborated in conducting a study and writing a revealing journal article for the medical community. This described their controlled double-blind investigation of reconstructive therapy used for the permanent elimination of low back pain. You will read about this in Chapter Six. In their article, Robert G. Klein, M.D. of Santa Barbara, California, William Kubitschek, D.O. of San Marcos, California, Andrew Kulik, D.O. of San Diego, California, and Thomas Dorman, M.D. of San Luis Obispo, California, included a back pain questionnaire. Using this questionnaire, most doctors are able to make a determination of the psychological involvement of the patient by his or her response to questions about physical limitations.

On your own, you might try this self-survey for making a subjective evaluation your personal backache problem or that of a loved one. Here is the physicians' back pain survey form that invariably helps to profile the extent of chronic low-back pain for the individual in agony:

BACK PAIN QUESTIONNAIRE

When your back hurts you may find it difficult to do some of the things you normally do. The list that follows contains some sentences that people have used to describe themselves when they have back pain. As you read them you may find that some statements stand out because they describe you the way you are today. Read the list and think of yourself today. When you read a sentence that describes how you are, put a check mark against it. If the sentence does not describe you, leave the space blank and go on to the next one. Remember to check off only the sentence if you are sure that it describes you as you are today. (Authors' notation: If you finish marking the survey form and notice that you have checked ten or more statements depicting the way you feel or behave today, it's likely that a reconstructive therapist will be helpful to you.) Here is the back pain questionnaire:

_____ I stay at home most of the time because of my back.
_____ I change position frequently to try and get my back comfortable.
_____ I walk more slowly than usual because of my back.
_____ I am not doing any of the jobs that I usually do around the house because of my back.
_____ I use a handrail to get up stairs because of my back.
_____ I lie down to rest more often because of my back.
_____ I have to hold on to something to get out of an easy chair because of my back.
_____ I try to get other people to do things for me because of my back.
_____ I get dressed more slowly than usual because of my back.

_____ I only stand up for short periods of time because of my back.

_____ I try not to bend or kneel down because of my back.

_____ I find it difficult to get out of a chair because of my back.

_____ My back is painful almost all of the time.

_____ I find it difficult to turn over in bed because of my back.

_____ My appetite is not very good because of my back pain.

_____ I have trouble putting on my socks (or stockings) because of the pain in my back.

_____ I only walk short distances because of my back pain.

_____ I sleep less well because of my back.

_____ I get dressed with help from someone else because of my back.

_____ I sit down for most of the day because of my back.

_____ I avoid heavy jobs around the house because of my back.

_____ I am more irritable and bad tempered with people than usual because of my back.

_____ I go upstairs more slowly than usual because of my back.

_____ I stay in bed most of the time because of my back.

A Case of Sciatica

Where the pain originates is another indication of its cause. However, the area of the pain may be misleading, as in the case of sciatica, a gnawing and constant burning-like twinge usually felt in the back of the thigh and down the legs, descending from the buttocks and often accompanied by numbness in the region of the ankle. When due to spinal root involvement, it is aggravated by change of posture, coughing, sneezing, or defecation. Joint, tendon, and ligament instability may also present these same sciatica-type of symptoms.

Sciatica-type pain was a condition affecting black-haired and brown-eyed Waukesha, Wisconsin housewife Katherine Honcharick, 45 years old, and newly married after a decade of widowhood. Sciatic neuritis had her feeling good for nothing — divorced from reality. She could not work as a volunteer in the Waukesha Memorial Hospital. She felt unable to sexually consummate her marriage to a new husband. Leg pain accompanied sexual foreplay and intercourse and was causing problems in her marriage. Additionally, this new wife could not do ordinary housework — the laundry, mop the floor, or even dust off the furniture.

Interviewing the woman on May 2, 1989, we were told, "My leg symptoms came from a herniated disk between two of the vertebrae of my spinal column. Besides sensations of gnawing ache down my left leg, I also felt sharpness and throbbing from my buttock all the way to the bottom of my foot. If I moved the wrong way, the sharp pains would shoot up and down. There were times that all I could do to get from room to room was crawl on the floor. I could not bear standing and putting weight on the leg. Oftentimes, all I did was lie on my bed with the phone by my head to keep in touch with the outside world. I couldn't go to the bathroom. I couldn't sit up; sitting was the most difficult position to maintain. I was very miserable with the constant burning pain. It continued from just after I got married, August 26, 1987, to January 6, 1989. I just tolerated living and lingered in constant agony almost this entire time. Then I got permanent relief from undergoing reconstructive therapy."

Before consulting Milwaukee pain specialist William J. Faber, D.O., Mrs. Honcharick took half-a-dozen cortisone shots, a month of physical therapy, daily hot packs and hot tubs at home, and she swallowed lots of pain pills prescribed by other doctors. "Nothing helped before," she said, "but now, after having three months of reconstructive therapy, I've returned to volunteer work at the hospital, push wheel chairs, bodily lift patients onto their beds, do all of my housework, go to the YWCA for aerobic exercise, and my husband is well satisfied in bed. Reconstructive therapy brought me back to being a whole person again."

As shown by two examinations from orthopedic surgeons and her computerized axial tomograph (CAT) scan, the source of Mrs. Honcharick's sciatica was a herniated disk at the fifth lumbar and first sacral vertebrae. A CAT scan is an established diagnostic radiological technique for the examination of the soft tissues of the body. It involves the recording of 'slices' of the body with an X-ray scanner; these records are then integrated by computer to give a cross-sectional image. The investigation is of minimal risk to the patient.

The last orthopedic surgeon that she visited wrote in his records: "Patient is to be scheduled for laminectomy the next time she calls." A herniated disk is the displaced position of a rounded flattened cartilaginous structure separating the bony vertebrae along the course of the spinal column. A laminectomy (also known as a rachiotomy) is the surgical cutting into the backbone to obtain access to the spinal cord. The surgeon removes the rear part (the posterior arch) of one or more vertebrae. The operation is performed to treat injuries to the spine, such as prolapsed intervertebral (slipped) disk (in which the affected disk is removed), or to relieve pressure on a spinal nerve. Mrs. Honcharick's scheduled laminectomy would have involved cutting into the backbone to obtain access to the spinal cord, as mentioned. The surgeon would then remove the rear part of one or more of her involved vertebrae, the fifth lumbar and first sacral.

Mrs. Honcharick would have been putting herself at risk. Many laminectomies fail, leaving the patient with an unstable spine, back stiffness, spinal arthritis, lack of endurance, and continuation of her sciatic pain.

Taking a structural part out of the body — a usual procedure during surgery — does not make the part that is left or the rest of the body stronger.

This is where reconstructive therapy has real advantage. Each treatment makes the structure stronger than before because it stimulates new tissue growth. Dr. Faber's proliferating injection solution and some manipulation procedures that he used allowed the patient to avoid laminectomy. It produced new tissue growth as ligamentous fibers. The injections began at once to build new ligament tissue. In three months Mrs. Honcharick found that her symptoms had completely disappeared, and they've not returned to this day.

NOTE TO HEALTH PROFESSIONALS: The case records of Waukesha, Wisconsin housewife Katherine Honcharick and all others cited here are available for viewing during preceptorship training in reconstructive therapy.

Building New Ligament Tissue

"The time has come," writes Martin H. Andrews, M.D. of Oklahoma City, Oklahoma, in an unpublished manuscript with the title Applications of Prolotherapy in Family Practice, "for a genuine and serious appraisal of the present dismal results of pharmacological, sensory (anesthetic blocking agents, low-level and high-level stimulation), psychological, and surgical efforts to relieve chronic pain. The [medical] profession needs to allow that impressive contributions are being made in the area of chronic pain treatment. The careful application of the principles of reconstructive therapy can, and does provide effective treatment; and acceptance of this modality need not, and should not exclude other approaches to chronic pain relief." In fact, Dr. Andrews' assertions are definitely being heeded by reconstructive therapists who are performing well for their patients by stimulating the formation of growth factors inside their damaged ligaments, tendons, and joints.

In the human body, growth factors are naturally occurring proteins that affect different parts of cells to promote new tissue growth. Others activate blood vessel regeneration. In particular, fibroblast growth factor works in the deeper layers of tissue to promote growth of tiny blood vessel cells and those that line the larger blood vessels, as well. These fibroblast growth factors stimulate the secretion of collagen — the weblike connective tissue that surrounds ligaments and all other tissue cells, especially skin cells.

"The promotion of more collagen growth is responsible for giving the healing tissue its tensile strength," says Dr. John Fiddles, vice president of research at California Biotechnology of Mountain View, California. This company, in 1985, began research to create synthetic proteins to speed wound healing. Other commercial research companies are engaged in developing new growth factors for the treatment of burns, surgical wounds, and various injuries. Mainly they are engaged in the search for proteins to build epidermal growth factors.[1]

Another protein, called platelet-derived growth factor, is drawing interest from researchers. It is believed to play a role similar to fibroblast growth factor in inducing fibroblasts to move into a wound (such as an injected ligament stimulated by proliferating solution) and build new connective tissue.

This is already being done in the offices and clinics of doctors who employ reconstructive therapy. The reconstruction therapists are stimulating the formation of natural growth factor at specific sites inside the human body, in particular at places where ligamentous injury has previously taken place. The therapy is proven beyond a shadow of a doubt to cause formation of new fibrous tissue in those injected with proliferating solutions.

**Animal Experiments that Prove the
Formation of New Ligaments**

"Animal experiments were reported in 1955 on the injection of a stimulating solution into the tendons of rabbits," reported Dr. George Hackett when he appeared before the Industrial Medicine Association's Annual Meeting in Atlantic City, New Jersey, in April, 1958. "[A study of the animals] revealed the stages of new fibrous tissue cellular growth throughout the tendon and new bone cellular growth at the fibro-osseous junction. The new tissue became permanent to strengthen the 'weld' of fibrous tissue to bone and explains the excellent results that have been obtained clinically." [2]

Dr. Hackett showed the assembly of industrial medicine physicians slides of the calf muscle tendons and superficial flexor tendons of the legs of rabbits which were treated with proliferating solution. The proliferant stimulated the production of permanent new bone and fibrous tissue cells at the fibro-osseous junction. Additional slides taken two months after the rabbits received their injections showed an abundance of fibrous ligament-like connection between the tendon and the fibrous bone matrix had been laid down. (See Figures 3 and 4 depicting the same photographs of rabbit tendons after proliferating solution had been administered to the animals.)

In a University of Iowa study, medial knee ligaments of rabbits were injected with 5 percent sodium morrhuate three times. As mentioned sodium morrhuate, a medication approved by the U.S. Food and Drug Administration (FDA), is purified from distilled cod liver oil. When the University of Iowa researchers tested the rabbits' ligaments, they found them to be permeated with the sodium morrhuate solution. The injected ligaments were 35 percent stronger in tensile strength and up to 40 percent larger in hypertrophied size than the noninjected control ligaments.

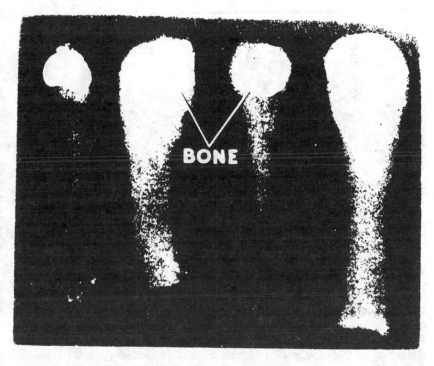

Figure 3. X-ray films of rabbit tendons made in 1958 by George S. Hackett, M.D. showing (on the extreme right) that injections with proliferants produce longer, thicker, and firmer tendon growth than the uninjected tendon (on the extreme left).

(Reprinted with permission from Hackett, G.S. Ligament and Tendon Relaxation Treated by Prolotherapy. Charles C. Thomas Publisher, Springfield, Illinois)

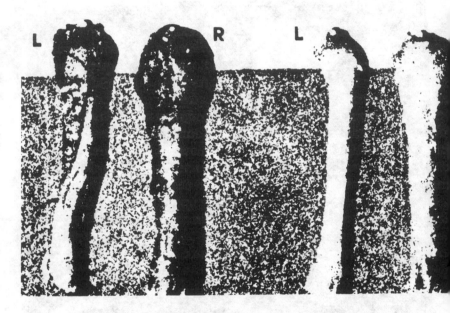

Figure 4. Rabbits tendons (marked "R") were injected with proliferants by George S. Hackett, M.D. three times. In contrast, other rabbit tendons (marked "L") were injected three times with only normal saline. The "R" tendons grew larger, thicker, and stronger by addition of 35-40 percent more tissue having increased weight and diameter.

(Reprinted with permission from Hackett, G.S. Ligament and Tendon Relaxation Treated by Prolotherapy. Charles C. Thomas Publisher, Springfield, Illinois)

Dr. Harold Walmer of Elizabethtown, Pennsylvania who has employed reconstructive therapy for his patients since 1952, believes that reconstructive therapy improves weakened ligaments in joint instability because of this ligament hypertrophy that results from the fibrous growth stimulation. Mildly irritating reconstructive solutions cause dilation of blood vessels with migration of fibroblasts to the injured areas. Fibroblasts lay down collagen for repair. This change is permanent. It was proven in further histologic studies of ligaments treated with a variety of proliferant solutions in the rabbit and rat. The ligaments demonstrated increases in ligament thickness, ligament mass of 20 to 40 percent, and in mass/length ratios.[3]

Then there were biomechanical measurements of ligament junction strength, using the rabbit medial collateral ligament as a model. The measurements show statistically significant increases in bone-ligament junction strength in treated animals (sodium morrhuate solution vs. saline solution) and controls. Then there was a 1988 live study in human knees using a series of intraligamentous dextrose-glycerine-phenol injections. These are proliferating solutions. The injections demonstrated significant increases in collateral ligament stability.[4]

Finally, the solutions employed to accomplish reconstructive therapy are proven by the Departments of Orthopaedic Surgery, Ostra Sjukhuset, Goteborg, Sweden and University of Iowa, Iowa City, Iowa, to mimic the injury-repair response in connective tissue. As described previously, the proliferants bring on "an early formation of granulation tissue, cellular hyperplasia, increases in water and amino sugar content, and a decrease in collagen fibril diameter and hydroxyproline content compared with control tendons. The decreased mean collagen fibril diameter appears to be due to the formation of new collagen fibrils as evidenced by an increased cell population and a more active appearing organelle network within the fibroblasts." The size of the newly formed fibrils is an increase in components of the tissue.[5]

Almost everyone who has impaired joints from damaged ligaments can benefit from receiving reconstructive therapy. But how do you know that you are a candidate for this treatment? How do you know that your investment of time, money, and short term discomfort will bring you the reward of no more chronic joint pain? Our next chapter offers you the answers to these questions.

Chapter Five

How to Know You Need Reconstructive Therapy

Now fifty-six years old, Charlie Roebuck of Kenosha, Wisconsin, a millwright in a Chrysler auto assembly plant, had been suffering with joint pain in the low back for over a decade. His troubles began with injury to his lumbosacral spine from an automobile accident. Roebuck is a hulk of a man, six feet tall and 230 pounds of bone, muscle, and gristle — a tough customer afraid of nothing and nobody. Before his accident he was occasionally known to knock heads together in Wisconsin beer halls. Soon that all changed because, as he described it, "The pain was awful. Lying down alone, I would turn my eyes to heaven and cry bitter tears. I pleaded with God, 'Oh, the pain — please stop it — Oh, it hurts. Pain, pain go away!' "

"That went on for more years than I care to recall, but it's different now. I'm cured of my back troubles, finally. Let me tell you what I went through then," said Roebuck, as he gestured with his big hands.

"When I bent down or turned in different ways I could feel pressure, soreness, and severe pain around the top of my hips and low down inside my spinal column," he reported when interviewed in March 1987. "I searched for medical help everywhere — from orthopedists, chiropractors, physical therapists, and several other types of health professionals. I took lots of drugs such as pain killers and muscle relaxants, went on rest cures, did exercises, wore braces, had cortisone shots, and underwent a disc surgery [laminectomy] eight years ago, and all the while I followed the many doctors' many directions.

"Treatment for me was to no avail. I still lived every day in misery. My back joints would pop, click, snap, and grind. I lacked strength and endurance. I stopped going into bar rooms for fear that I'd get in a fight that I couldn't handle. My joints had stiffness and aches. A new brace helped for a time and then stopped doing me any good. Visits to my chiropractor for back adjustments felt fine for a while and then the effect disappeared by the time I woke up the next day," continued Charlie Roebuck. "I had to rest lots to get any kind of relief. The laminectomy did me no good at all — just added to my overall stress. I could stand or walk for only about 40 minutes and then would have to get some rest. Lying flat on my back on the floor provided me with the best position for pain relief. Even driving in the car was impossible because of bumps in the road that jarred my body. Whereas in the past I could lift one end of an 800-pound steel rod so as to carry it to the workbench, I found myself unable even to hold fifty pounds because of penetrating back pain. I slept poorly and woke up fatigued — always feeling that I needed toothpicks to hold open my eyelids. Cortisone injections that I received helped not at all. I was in a hell of a mess."

Then another back patient referred Roebuck to the Milwaukee Pain Clinic where the clinic's medical director, osteopathic physician Dr. William J. Faber, made the correct diagnosis and administered reconstructive therapy. Dr. Faber, trained in the administration of biological medicine and the elimination of the causes of pain, applies therapeutic methods that are considerably different and often far more effective than standard allopathic-orthopedic surgery for an impaired musculoskeletal system. We will return to Charlie Roebuck later in this chapter, but for now you should know the concepts behind his reconstruction treatment and eventual recovery.

Biological Method Vs Medicine/Surgery Method of Joint Treatment

In the biological method of joint treatment (see Figure 5), a physician intending to administer reconstructive therapy has certain goals in mind for his or her patient's body structure. First, the doctor desires to aid the patient's immune system and natural healing ability. Second, he/she wants to stimulate a kind of controlled inflammation, because inflammation is the body's first step in healing.

Inflammation is a reaction of the body tissues and blood circulation to injury, irritation, and infection. The biologically-minded physician attempting to correct a dysfunctioning joint with reconstructive therapy produces an immediate defensive reaction of body tissue by injecting the proliferating chemical or nutrient. The injection may bring on heat, redness, swelling, and local irritation. Blood vessels near the site become dilated, so blood flow is locally increased. Greater nourishment to the connective tissue of impaired ligaments causes strengthening and restoration of normal function by creation of new connective tissue called "cicatrix."

Thus biological methods of joint treatment differ very much from the allopathic techniques of American organized medicine. Biological methods cause the body's healing mechanism to undertake permanent natural reconstructions of joint structures. Not so the medicine/surgery method of joint treatment employed by allopathic physicians (see Figure 6). In contrast, their goals are to block pain with sedatives, narcotics, anti-inflammatory agents, and other pain killers, just the opposite from reconstructing physicians. They surgically remove torn and roughened tissue structures, including bone, ten-

BIOLOGICAL METHOD OF JOINT TREATMENT

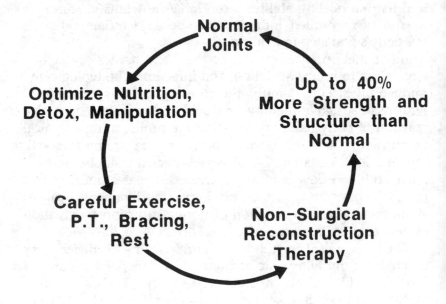

Figure 5. The biological method of joint treatment achieves two goals. (1) It aids the body's healing process. (2) It stimulates controlled inflammation so that the natural healing mechanism brings on permanent structural reconstruction for joint stabilization.

THE MEDICINE/SURGERY METHOD OF JOINT TREATMENT

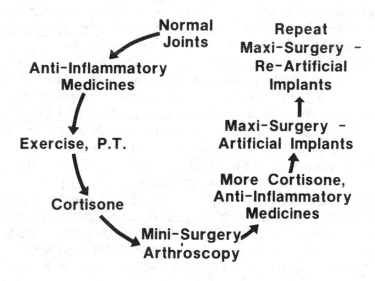

Figure 6. In the medicine/surgery method of joint treatment, contrary goals are sought: (1) block pain, (2) block inflamation, (3) remove torn, frayed or roughened structures, and (4) replace with artificial parts.

dons, and ligaments. Then they attempt to substitute artificial parts for the natural components of the body which entails additional major surgery. In acute fractures, total ruptures of tendons and ligaments, and some other conditions, surgery may be required.

The Technique of Reconstructive Therapy

A long, slender needle much like the acupuncturist's tool is used to place a stimulating solution in exactly the right place — where the ligament attaches into the bone. Sodium morrhuate, a typical solution, is a United States Food and Drug Administration-approved substance purified from distilled cod liver oil. It has been used in medicine extensively as a sclerotherapeutic agent for esophageal varices, varicose veins, hernia repair without surgery, obliteration of hemorrhoids, and possibly for other tissue-correction purposes. When it is combined in a syringe with the anesthetic procaine (changed by the human body into the B vitamin para-aminobenzoic acid, PABA) and a natural antihistamine, it causes controlled irritation. This causes your body to send healing cells (fibroblasts) to bring about a natural repair in the injected ligamentous attachments of the joint. Sodium morrhuate, however, is just one of perhaps 100 different solutions that are quite useful in reconstructive therapy.

When the needle tip touches the patient's bone at the joint site, the operator pulls back slightly or stays right on the bone. The amount of solution injected can be from a tenth to a whole cc or more. The injection is given tightly and firmly.

In two or three minutes, the anesthetic agent brings relief of pain. Procaine's anesthetic effect lasts from four to six hours. The sodium morrhuate then slowly excites the local cells into undergoing their process of repair and healing. It causes fibrous tissue to begin growing so that torn ligaments and tendons proliferate with new substance. This tissue proliferation comes from the local irritation-producing inflammation. Redness, heat, and swelling, and even some pain may come about from an influx of blood to the affected area. Fluid known as lymph causes more swelling of the affected tissues, compressing the nerve endings and thus producing slight pain. There may be temporary loss of function. A knee joint, for instance, may become stiff for a day or two and sometimes longer.

Each treatment causes the patient's own connective tissue to add on and strengthen formerly unstable joints, discs, and cartilage. Depending on the severity and location of disability, the number of reconstruction sessions required vary from six to thirty or more. At the Milwaukee Pain Clinic and Metabolic Research Center, 50 or more series of injections have been administered to individual patients for total spinal reconstruction. Total body reconstruction in some patients can require multiple sets of injections — perhaps even as many as a hundred. Dr. Faber has never witnessed recurrences of the original problems in a reconstructed area because the area becomes stronger than normal. He reports that four of his patients have experienced car accidents after their joint reconstructions in the back were completed. Although they injured the very areas that had been reconstructed, none of these patients had any resumption of their back symptoms.

Both authors have taken multiple sets of injections with proliferants for their individual joint problems. As with the many physicians who have taken reconstructive therapy themselves and also participated in the writing of this book by their contributing case histories and other information for this book, we have benefited markedly by receiving the treatment.

Body Detoxification Is Very Important
for Joint Reconstruction

If the patient feels that his treatment is beneficial, it is continued. If he shows no improvement or gets worse, the biological therapist does an indepth evaluation of the patient's biochemistry. How the physiological processes are functioning is a major factor in the success of reconstructive therapy. For example, defecation must be large, frequent, and regular; digestion has to be comfortable and steady; heavy metals must not be contaminating the body, including silver dental amalgams (both Dr. Faber and Dr. Walker have had their silver dental amalgams removed from their teeth and replaced them with gold or composite materials); the yeast syndrome can't be bringing on symptoms of immune suppression, etc. The injection technique will be discontinued until the patient's physiology is in good shape. Body detoxification is illustrated by Figures 7, 8, and 9.

Figure 7 depicts the body as a beaker containing the accumulated products of metabolism. As the body functions and uses up nutrients, it gives off waste products that are stored for eventual disposal. If disposal does not take place on a frequent and regular basis, or wastes are allowed to gather because of some pathological blockage to the bowel, urinary tract, skin, lymphatics, blood circulation, lungs or other system, the person falls into a state of subclinical illness. He thinks, "I'm fine! There's nothing wrong with me." But he is getting ready to manifest symptoms and signs of disease. The straws are building up. The individual's body is reaching the point of intolerance to accumulated wastes.

Figure 8 depicts the body exceeding its tolerance of waste product accumulation so that it spills over with signs of illness. The patient thinks, "Oh, I got sick all of a sudden." Not true! He or she did not get sick suddenly. Rather, the person earned his or her illness. He or she drank soda pop, allowed yeast overgrowth, harbored chronic viral infections, failed to eat vegetables, smoked cigarettes, and did other things to make the body ill.

A state of
"OKness" is
present when
toxic load is
contained with-
in the body's
storage areas.
No overt symp-
oms are noticed.

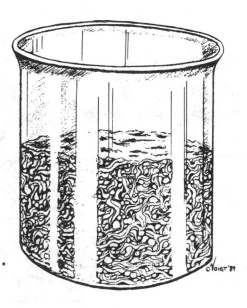

Figure 7. The human body may be depicted by a beaker holding toxins. The individual with these toxins feels no symptoms, although he or she suffers from subclinical illness or a predisease status.

Toxic load capacity is exceeded with resulting symptoms and illness present.

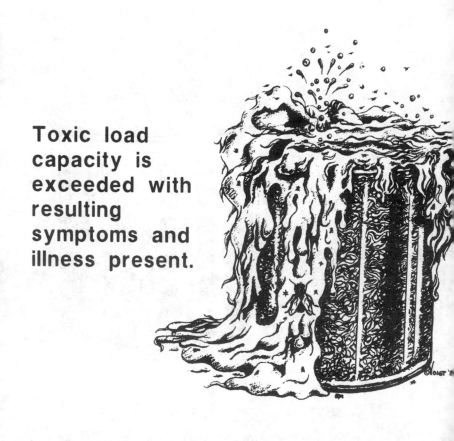

Figure 8. When the body's ability, depicted as a beaker, is exceeded it spills over with symptoms and signs of illness.

**A clean body
has no toxins
and optimal
healing ability.**

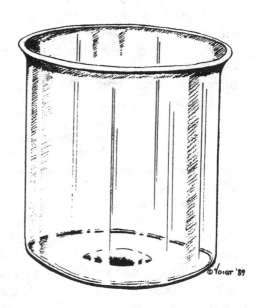

Figure 9. Keeping the body free of toxins will keep it free of illness.

Figure 9 depicts that a body detoxified — a body totally clean — has no germs, the absence of degenerations, and a defense system that is working perfectly. A really healthy person gets no colds, feels no aches and pains, has no allergies, and experiences no downtime. Why? Because he or she detoxifies the body on a regular basis. Significant to this concept of detoxification is that cancer, a multifactural disease related to toxicity, was present, in 1900, in three out of 100 Americans. It grew in number to one out of seven by World War II. In the 1980's, it increased to one out of three.

A knowledgeable mechanic or automotive engineer will tell you that you can keep an automobile running for a hundred years. But to do this, you must optimize the car's condition. Don't wait until you need to call a tow truck. The same applies to a human body. The failure to detoxify means you are waiting for the crisis.

The University of Iowa Study on Laboratory Animals

With biological therapy, the Arndt-Schultz Law applies. This law states that small stresses are stimulating, and large stresses seem to inhibit stimulation. The Arndt-Schultz law is illustrated by a small electrical current such as the TENS current which stimulates circulation and healing in bones. On the other hand, a large electrical current such as the electric chair decreases circulation and results in death. So it is with the biological methods used in reconstructive therapy. The mildly irritating reconstructive solutions cause dilation of blood vessels and migration of fibroblasts to the injured areas. Fibroblasts lay down collagen for repair. This change appears to be permanent and is measurable by an increased potential for ligamentous structures (see Figure 10). Of course, periodic application of proliferants may become necessary after the patient reaches recovery to maintain the ligaments' and tendons' optimal level of strength and function, particularly if

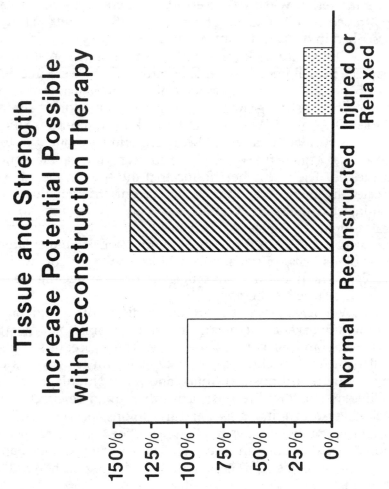

Figure 10. Tissue and strength can be measured for normal, damaged, and reconstructed ligaments.

anatomy has been lost or removed.

Harold Walmer, D.O. of Elizabethtown, Pennsylvania has been an advocate of reconstructive therapy since 1952. He became interested when he observed the increased white areas of X-rayed rabbit tendons of Dr. George S. Hackett's study[1] (described in detail in Chapter Four).

In a University of Iowa study[2] (also described in the last chapter), medial knee ligaments of other rabbits were injected with 5 percent sodium morrhuate three times. The excellent ligamentous tissue growth occurring in the rabbits so intrigued Dr. Harold Walmer that he took up the serious study of reconstructive therapy and became a prime exponent of the procedure. Ligaments were removed from the rabbit bones and tested. The researchers found that the sodium morrhuate injected ligaments were almost 40 percent stronger than the non-injected ones. Dr. Walmer has stated in lectures to his professional colleagues that it is this ligament hypertrophy — the increase in size of the tissue brought about by the enlargement of its cells, plus possible cellular multiplication within the ligament fibers that accounts for patients feeling better after reconstructive therapy.

Dr. Walmer believes that reconstruction with proliferants improves weakened ligments in joint instability of nearly every type and all parts of the body. The procedure is particularly useful in chronic low back pain, unstable knees or ankles due to arthritis or trauma, and other chronic joint disability. He has found reconstructive therapy to be effective in such diverse conditions as painful bunions, plantar fasciitis, temporomandibular dysfunction of the jaw, recurrent shoulder dislocation, and nearly all other joint, tendon, and ligament problems regardless of the severity or duration of the problem.

Charlie Roebuck Permanently Gets Rid
of Pain in His Lumbar Spine

Having his experience with the biological method of reconstructive therapy, Charlie Roebuck found that he benefitted tremendously. He already had gone through his fill of allopathic medicine/surgery failure, and now he finally found something that really worked. Dr. Faber's biological procedure corrected dysfunction in Roebuck's skeletal system by restoring strength, increasing endurance, and stimulating self-repair of ligaments, tendons, and joints.

After his laboratory and clinical examinations of the patient, including an x-ray evaluation at the Milwaukee-based Northwest General Hospital by certified radiologist Thomas Roskos, M.D., D.O., Dr. Faber decided that Roebuck would markedly gain from reconstruction therapy and proceeded to bring the treatment to completion for him.

When interviewed about two-and-a-half years ago, the man had already taken eight injection treatments. He said then, "The injections have improved my life altogether. Unlike before the treatments, now I can turn in any direction without pain in my lumbar spine. At work, I lift heavy steel plates at Chrysler and pay them no mind. I can take long walks — even run — when before, as I told you, chronic back soreness, aching, and pulling sensations would cause me to sit down or lie down at any opportunity. My increased activity alone has let me drop twelve pounds of excess weight in seven weeks. I just don't feel joint pain in my back anymore."

When interviewed again in August 1989, Charlie Roebuck reported that ten reconstruction injections were all that he needed for total and absolute relief. After that, he felt cured. And Dr. Faber affirmed that he could discontinue treatment. Roebuck's back has been perfectly fine — no discomfort whatsoever — since his last injection, he reports. Except for being uncomfortable at the time of injection and stiffness with swelling at the injection site for a day or two, there were no noticeable side effects, Roebuck said.

"In fact," he stated with a smile, "the reconstructive therapy seemed only to have an overriding good side effect — less pain and eventually no pain ever again in my back."

When the treated area becomes firmer and stronger in a week or so, as is usual, the doctor using reconstruction treatment need not even ask if the patient feels less pain. The doctor knows this to be the case by seeing and feeling greater tone in the patient's tissues.

How to Know You're a Candidate
for Reconstructive Therapy

Charlie Roebuck lost the pain in his back and it felt stronger, firmer, more stable, and had greater tissue tone. His clinician's goal was to produce optimum solidness in any joints causing the patient discomfort. The man spent a long and unnecessarily painful time before finally receiving reconstructive therapy. When he did, it was a most gratifying experience. Still, it was too bad that he had not known how to recognize that he was a prime candidate for the treatment. He had nearly all of the classic signs and symptoms that pointed the way.

So how do you know that the treatment is for you? In the end, only the trained physician/therapist is able to make that therapeutic decision. Doctors with no training or experience in reconstructive therapy simply are unqualified. (In the section following this, we will explain about how a physician can receive training in joint reconstruction.) However, as a potential patient, your answers of "yes" to several of the following questions most likely mean that you could benefit by having this reconstructive injection treatment:

_____ Do you take anti-inflammatory drugs such as aspirin,

cortisone, Motrin™, Nuprin™, Nalfon™, Clinoril™, Feldene™, Naprosyn™,Indocin™, Tolectin™, or the equivalent, for relieving shoulder joint pain, tennis elbow, chronic ankle sprain, migraine headache, bursitis, foot trouble such as heel spurs, neuritis, arthritis, tendonitis, backache, chronic stiff neck, or another type of musculoskeletal disorder?

_____ Do you have a joint that makes sounds — grindings, pops, clicks, or snaps?

_____ Do you lack strength and endurance because of chronic joint pain?

_____ Do you have symptoms of arthritis with accompanying general joint discomforts of stiffness, ache, pain, more grinding sounds, and/or disquieting inflammation?

_____ Do you now feel joint discomfort or have you experienced the presence of synovitis, tendonitis, or another musculoskeletal problem for longer than six weeks?

_____ Do you find you need some aid for an uncomfortable body part from the use of a brace, splint, or supportive strapping?

_____ Do you experience quick comfort from chiropractic adjustment or osteopathic manipulation but are soon disappointed by discovering that the professional treatment does not last?

_____ Do you find no lasting relief from massage, manipulationacupressure, *shiatsu*, reflexology, adjustments, myotherapy, Rolfing, the Feldenkrais technique, polarity therapy, orgone therapy, Alexander technique, Bio-Energetics, Mensendieck System, Lotte Berk Method, or another form of manual body work?

_____ Do you feel greater joint comfort with rest and worse joint discomfort after exercise (except swimming and bicycling)?

_____ Have you undergone surgery wherein natural joint spacers such as discs, menisci, or other cartilagenous structures have been removed but pain is still present?

_____ Have you undergone surgery for correction of tendons, hip replacement, ligaments, carpal tunnel syndrome, spinal fusion or pinning, herniated disc, fractures, chronic joint dislocation, or other surgery and still experience pain?

_____ Are you able to stand, sit, or walk for only a half hour or less and then have to change position?

_____ If you rest in one position for a time, such as lying on your back, do you feel compelled to change position relatively soon because of pain, pressure sense, or other discomforts?

_____ Do bumps in the road while you are riding in an automobile increase your pain?

_____ Does lifting 30 pounds or more of weight increase your pain?

_____ Do you have swelling or aching in a body part after use or after exercise?

_____ Have cortisone injections or nerve injections failed to help relieve your pain or helped for just a short while?

_____ Do you sleep poorly, frequently awaken during the night, change bed positions often, wake up with a headache, or feel pain in a body part upon arising?

_____ Do you find difficulty getting out of a chair, walking down stairs, or rolling in bed from your abdomen to your back?

_____ Do you feel that your knee, shoulder, back, or another body part just snap out of position or otherwise go out on you?

Interpreting the Indications

Knowing that ligaments and tendons stabilize a joint by

holding its bones in place provides a means of interpreting the signs and symptoms that may indicate you are a candidate for reconstruction therapy. You should realize that when ligaments are torn or extremely loose as a result of sudden trauma or from wear and tear, they are unable to effectively perform their jobs. Your body attempts to correct the ligaments' laxness and resulting joint instability by bringing osteoblasts (bone-forming cells) to the area. The osteoblasts lay down extra (metastatic) bone to act as a splint. Medical scientists refer to this pathologic splinting as "arthritis." Thus, arthritis is the body's attempt to compensate for your weakened ligaments' inability to hold the joint's bones in position. Additionally, the muscles go into spasm to help support the weakened joint. The muscles are not the primary problem, although their spasming hurts along with the inflamed and arthritic joint. Reconstructive therapy permanently corrects this arthritic condition. It is the opposite to the destruction of tissue resulting from cortisone injections, which dissolve fibrous structures, soften bones, and produce metabolic imbalances.

Reconstructing the soft tissue surrounding a joint means that there is a building up and laying down of new connective substances so that excessive joint movement stops. The ligaments, tendons, and joints are restored to good health. They more fully perform their functions of support and stabilization. It's not proven but assumed from clinical results that osteoblasts disengage from their local bone-producing processes and joint-splinting terminates. Thus, bone grinding and joint snapping sounds known as "crepitus" no longer are heard. Simultaneously, inflammation with its pain and swelling goes away. The symptoms of arthritis in the joint are gone forever when the joint is fully reconstructed. Joint pain goes away, not to return.

The Doctor's Training and Skill with Reconstructive Therapy

The biologic procedure we are discussing must be carried out by a physician trained, tested, and skilled in the use of reconstructive therapy. Such training is given by the American Osteopathic Academy of Sclerotherapy, Inc., in seminar form. Telephone for training information from the American Osteopathic Association at (800) 621-1773. Training in the form of a preceptorship is given, as well, by Dr. William Faber to interested physicians who spend considerable concentrated study time as preceptors at the Milwaukee Pain Clinic and Metabolic Research Center, 6529 West Fond du Lac Avenue, Milwaukee, Wisconsin 53218. Telephone (414) 464-PAIN or (414) 464-7680.

The Milwaukee Pain Clinic preceptor program involves practical application of the injection procedures themselves, along with the principles of the biologic method. Physician preceptorship training allows dedicated M.D.s and D.O.s to rapidly learn the skills, procedures, and ideas necessary to master this treatment. Furthermore, physicians receive training in neural therapy, a break-through German-derived nerve and loss-of-range-of-motion corrective technique using procaine or lidocaine injections. It provides instant subjective and objective therapeutic results. (Watch for a new book by the authors about this remarkable therapy called *Instant Relief from Pain and Dysfunction.*

The preceptor program welcomes osteopathic (D.O.) and allopathic (M.D.) physicians for a hands-on education with responding patients under physician-teacher supervision. The course covers the complexities of injection technique and solution selection, safety procedures, patient benefits to be anticipated, diagnosis, contraindications, possible side effects, prognosis, and more. All of the previous preceptors have gone back to their clinics to employ the teachings and reported exciting results for their patients. None have reported any adverse or unexpected reactions. This course of instruction at the Milwaukee Pain Clinic is in the process of being certified by the American Academy of Neurological and Orthopaedic Surgeons.

Reconstructive therapy presents a win-win situation for the patients and their doctors. There is no single therapeutic procedure which can match its permanent healing benefits.

James Carlson, D.O. of Knoxville, Tennessee and Kent Pomeroy, M.D. of Phoenix, Arizona, both former presidents of the American Association of Orthopaedic Medicine, say: "No physician and surgeon, regardless of training, should attempt to administer reconstructive therapy from reading this book or from any book or journal articles on the method. Physicians only trained by specific preceptorship are qualified to safely apply the treatment. Serious complications, paralysis, even death from inadvertently using incorrect technique, could occur. These have been reported from a reaction to the treatment rendered by inexperienced hands. Sodium morrhuate and other biological proliferants can be extremely potent and produce adverse reactions." In contrast, Rodney Chase, D.O. of Bethlehem, Pennsylvania states that reconstructive therapy when administered by a knowledgeable and skilled physician is safer than giving an injection of cortisone.

Because of the potential for side effects or contraindications connected with reconstructive therapy, the coauthors and their publisher disclaim any form of liability as a result of you or anyone else using the information in this book. Information that is published here does not substitute for the medical advice and supervision of your personal physician. No medical therapy should be undertaken except under the direction of a physician or other health professional from whom you seek advice.

Chapter Six

Backache and How to End It

French Canadian policeman Claude Linette, fifty-eight years old, told us that nine years ago he could no longer face the prospect of continuing life because of the pain in his back. The intense aching he had endured for over 21 years was driving him to suicide. He decided to throw himself into a line of traffic at an opportune moment while on the job.

His pain, ache, stress, sleeplessness, depression, anxiety, and other discomforts related to his back trouble had begun in 1960 when he was directing traffic in downtown Toronto. He was hit first by a car and then by a bus coming from the other direction. Unconscious, he was taken to the hospital in an ambulance, where he lingered between life and death for almost a week. He had broken arms, leg, collarbone, and ribs, and crushing injury to the spine. Moved from intensive care to a private room, he thought he was lucky to have survived. His arms, leg, collarbone, and four broken ribs healed fine. Until his full-body cast came off, he thought that he would have no residual effect from the trauma. Getting out of bed on what was to have been his wedding day, he was struck by such a sharp back pain that he was thrown to his knees and then onto his back on the floor. The pain was so deep, stabbing, and persistent that he couldn't crawl to the call button. Trying to get up only brought on greater agony. He had to lie on the floor until his friend and best man happened to come by to check on him.

Diagnostic procedures determined that Officer Linette had

sustained ruptured intervertebral discs in both the thoracic (dorsal bulge behind the chest) and lumbar (lumbar bulge behind the loins) of the back. Eight back bones were involved, and it seemed that the young officer's promising career in the police department was going to be abbreviated or, at least, much limited.

Pain killers hardly brought any comfort. Paid for by Canadian socialized medicine, the Toronto Police Department authorized Claude to have a laminectomy for removal of the rear portions of all of the affected vertebrae. As described in the case history of Katherine Honcharick in Chapter Four, laminectomy is the surgical removal of the rear arch of a vertebra to relieve pressure on the spinal cord. Such pressure was believed to be the cause of Officer Linette's severe pain.

The patient spent two months recovering from his surgical ordeal and then found that the pain continued anyway. He just had to bear it and maintain himself on prescribed medications, the orthopedic surgeon said. He did as best he could. He went back to work even though he was hurting, and it took everything he could muster.

Then while he was on night duty and checking on the roof of a bank, a thiry-foot ladder he was climbing slipped and threw Claude 35 feet onto some garbage cans. Again he was hospitalized for several weeks. He returned to police work, but his back pain hit again with a fury. It forced him to take additional time for convalescence. He would lie in bed or flat on the floor at home moaning. He felt good for nothing — absolutely useless.

Claude's wife apparently felt the same, for she finally told him that if he did not find some kind of permanent medical help and get the problem taken care of she would leave him. With this warning ringing in his ears, the man desperately sought more orthopedic care. The new orthopedist immediately put the patient into the hospital and strung him up in

71

traction. He lay stretched out for three weeks with no appreciable improvement. Strong pain killers were mandatory just to help him hold back tears brought on by the severe pain.

Out of a sense of failure, the second orthopedic surgeon referred Claude to a neurosurgeon who performed another laminectomy. Again the patient lingered in a hospital for weeks and recuperated at home for another month. When he did not show improvement, the neurosurgeon ordered that a myelogram be carried out. The young fellow underwent still a third laminectomy. He practically had no whole backbones left in his lumbar spinal areas.

The orthopedist, the neurosurgeon, and a variety of internists and other specialists that had been brought in as consultants then told Officer Linette that they had done all they could. There was no more bone to be removed from his back, they said, and he could now expect to slowly become paralyzed. He lay in bed for another month determined that paralysis was not going to be his fate. So, after his back had healed sufficiently, Officer Linette returned to night patrol down Toronto's back streets.

The fellow tried to help himself. He started wearing a back brace. He went through daily physical therapy. Chiropractic treatment gave him some short term relief. He joined a health club and exercised each day, too. In six months of trying to give his body a lift, he suffered severely while on the job, but found that he could hold off surrendering to the pain long enough to finish a work shift. By the end of eight hours on the job, he had to rush home and go to bed because of the pain.

Time passed. The chiropractic adjustments finally stopped helping. Pain pills never came near to giving relief. The exercises started to cause more discomfort than they alleviated. The police department's orthopedic surgeon was able to offer no solution. Claude later learned that the orthopedist had told

72

the Chief of Police that there was no reason he could discern for this young man to complain of pain. The Chief decided that Claude was a bad influence on the rest of the department, so work details became more difficult for him.

Claude transferred to a desk job where he found the situation somewhat easier. Then a chair collapsed under his weight. His fellow officers had a good laugh at his expense, but this accident only served to exacerbate the back trouble. He suffered more. Pain penetrated his entire being from his spinal area outward. His wife started to give him difficulty again, as well, because she wanted babies, and Claude found himself unable to perform sexually. He also didn't believe that he could continue in his position as a policeman and support a family. Besides, another idea was growing in his mind — a means of escaping his pain forever. He was determined to transfer to the traffic division again so as to be in a position to kill himself and have his widow collect compensation from the city.

That transfer took place in 1980. He was nearly prepared for suicide, when, at a social occasion, Claude happened to meet Jean-Paul Ouilette, M.D. of Orleans, Ontario Canada. Dr. Ouilette is a reconstruction therapist — one of the most skilled in Ontario Province. From their informal discussions, Claude became persuaded to try for relief just one more time, before he took the final way out. Dr. Ouilette applied reconstructive therapy to Claude's back. Upon receiving a series of injections, life for the policeman turned around altogether. The policeman states that now, nine years later, he is able to work everyday and to do all the activities that are demanded of him. He has no more pain. He is still married to the same woman and the father of two children. He is a sergeant on the Toronto Police Traffic Squad. Claude Linette says that if it were not for reconstructive therapy and Dr. Jean-Paul Ouilette, he would be dead today.

The Incidence of Backache

Back pain is sometimes regarded as more of a joke than a serious health problem, and a subject of folklore rather than medical science. Yet back disease is the cause of personal disability, much mental anguish, inability to work, deteriorating lifestyles, drop in income, and loss of personal relationships. Back pain doesn't kill, but it makes its victims wish they were dead.

As readily as it strikes a steel worker or a truck driver, backache has attacked Elizabeth Taylor, Jack Nicklaus, the late John F. Kennedy, and thousands of other celebrities. Nor is it confined to the old and infirm. The peak age at which backache comes on is between 35 and 45, but it is so universal that four out of five people will have back trouble at some time in their lives. Even if you've been lucky enough to escape so far, sooner or later, you're likely to become part of the backache brigade.

Throughout the world, millions of sufferers of back pain — especially in Western industrialized countries — are making huge demands on medical resources at a time when the cost of medical care is escalating. In Great Britain today, for instance, 56,000 people stay home from work each day because of back pain, and most face a loss of income in addition to the discomfort they experience. Since the average spell of absence from work lasts six weeks, the English taxpayer picks up an annual bill for almost 20 million days of sickness benefit. In Canada, another country with government welfare-type medicine, the annual taxpayer cost for its population's backaches alone is 9.2 million days of sickness benefit. For the United States each year, backache among 18 million of its citizens reduces the country's gross national product by $85 billion.

It seems almost incredible that a health problem that affects about 80 percent of the world's people has so long gone without an established cure. Current uncertainty about the most successful forms of treatment aggravate the difficulties of permanently correcting back complaints. All too frequently sufferers report a bewildering succession of ineffective therapies. Much of the medical community knows almost as little about effective mechanisms of care for back pain as when our caveman ancestors injured their spines rolling rocks to keep dinosaurs at bay. The back pain victim who does not respond to drugs, physiotherapy, traction, or bed rest may be referred by the primary care physician to any number of different types of specialists — a rheumatologist, an orthopedist, a neurosurgeon, a gynecologist, a urologist, an internist, a general surgeon or, if all else fails, to a psychiatrist.

In fact, the most effective treatment for your backache — reconstructive therapy — has been overlooked by nearly all health care practitioners. Among the reasons for this oversight is that the pharmaceutical industry and medical equipment manufacturers have no interest in promoting the therapy. There is no huge profit in it for them. The solutions used for injection in reconstructive therapy are not under patent, so the price cannot be marked up to support vigorous promotion and advertising.

The reconstruction injection technique reverses back pain by permanently correcting intravertebral ligament tears and stabilizing spinal subluxation. Proliferative agents are useful for reversing the pain of cervical, lumbar, thoracic, and sacral backaches. Reconstructive therapy has gone unappreciated too long when it has tremendous value for those desperate, depressed, and hopeless millions who suffer chronic back pain.

Why do these problems come on us? Why do four fifths of the people in the western world have chronic back trouble? Why is the back so predisposed to trauma and disease? Why, in fact, is backache one of the commonest of all physical complaints? One need merely take a close look at the human spinal column to know the answers to all of these questions.

Simplified Anatomy of the Spine

Most anthropologists agree that when evolution produced the human erect posture it also provided the cause of many backaches. Temporary backache may follow overexertion as when shoveling snow or moving furniture, or it may be a symptom of an acute illness such as influenza. Such simple troubles are not the kind of backache we are talking about. The anatomical arrangement of the spinal column gives rise to far more complicated difficulties than these. Reconstructive therapy takes the most serious back disability and corrects it effectively, quickly, and permanently.

The human spine resembles a spring, curved like the letter S. It has four bulges. The top cervical bulge in the neck region is forward, as is the lumbar bulge in the loin region. The dorsal bulge in the thoracic region curves backward, as does the sacral bulge in the lower back.

As a man or woman gets older, the spine loses its flexibility and tends to form an arch instead of a spring. The shoulders become stooped and the lumbar curve is reduced and turns the wrong way. Consquently, backaches become more common with advancing years.

The spinal column is composed of 24 separate bones called vertebrae, and two fused bones: the sacrum (five fused vertebrae) and the coccyx (four fused vertebrae). The vertebrae are separated from each other by cushions (or shock absorbers) made of cartilage called intervertebral discs. The discs are held tightly in place by strong ligaments such as the broad and flat innerspinous ligaments in an undamaged neck (see Figure 11) and the strong and firm ligaments between the spinous processes of the vertebrae in the low back (see Figure 12). Displacement of the discs in the lumbar or loin region be-

76

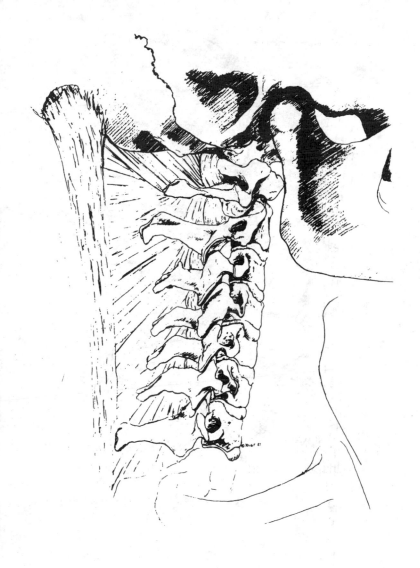

Figure 11. Ligaments of a normal neck (showing the broad stabilizing innerspinous tissues).

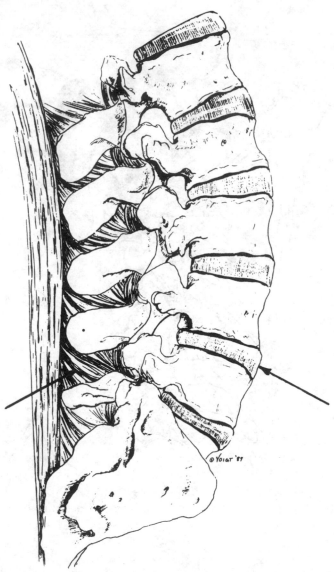

Figure 12. *Ligaments of the normal low back with correct disc heights and taut stabilizing tissues.*

cause of weak, overly lax, or torn ligaments is the commonest cause of persistent backaches.

A vertebra is shaped like a ring, with the main body in front, a wing (transverse process) on either side, and a projection (spinous process) behind. The spinal cord passes through the ring and the spinal nerves emerge from the notches (foramina) between each pair of vertebrae.

Besides the bones of the spine, tendons at the ends of the muscles of the back are also vulnerable. Tendons of two big muscles — the Trapezius (shaped like a trapezium) above and the Latissiumus dorsi (broadest tendon of the back) below — may cause a backache when strained by severe overexertion.

Certain occupations — which impose more stress upon the spinal column than it can tolerate, particularly in the loin or lumbar region — may predispose people to backaches. Men required to lift heavy freight are common sufferers, as are ballet dancers (who twist and turn their bodies into graceful but contorted positions). Chauffeurs who sit all day, and dentists and hairdressers who stand all day — tilting their bodies forward to work on the mouth or hair — are prone to suffer from backaches. A traffic officer such as Claude Linette who stands on hard pavement may lose a full inch in height during his workday as a result of the powerful but often overlooked forces of gravity. A good night's rest permits his flexible spine to spring back and the lost inch is restored.

If the legs are of unequal length — after tuberculosis or arthritis of the hip, operations for these conditions, or fracture of the neck of the femur (thighbone) near the hip joint — the whole body is thrown off balance and an inordinate effort by the spine and its ligaments and tendons and muscles is required to maintain correct posture. Sometimes musculoskeletal surgery causes as many problems as it is meant to correct.

The causes of backache may be classified as extrinsic (originating outside the spinal column) and intrinsic (originating in the spinal column).

There are many extrinsic causes, including systemic infections, diseases of the nervous system, malfunction of the parathyroid gland, displacement of the uterus in pregnancy, adhesions and scars following abdominal surgery, and metastases of cancer to the spine. To this list may be added obesity and flat feet. Contrary to popular belief, backache does not usually indicate a kidney disease.

The principal intrinsic causes of persistent backaches include displaced intervertebral discs, sprain and strain of ligaments and tendons, sacroiliac arthritis, and rheumatoid arthritis of the lower spine.

The most common cause of back trouble, however, is some sort of trauma — sudden or repetitive — an accident or awkward movement (such as may occur in assemblyline work, riding horseback, playing golf, pressing a foot pedal, etc.). Movements that tear the ligaments that hold discs in place and allow them to slip outside and press on the spinal nerves, causing pain, are chief among the causes of backache. Several decades ago a popular dance, well named as the twist, dislocated a lot of discs and brought on severe back aches. The symptoms of slipped disc are called low backache, lumbago, or sciatica, depending on the degree of dislocation and the amount of pressure on the sciatic and other nerves emerging from the spinal column.

The reconstruction therapist is able to palpate the back and determine the site of a weakened joint with its possible disc dislocation. In other cases, an x-ray is required to make the exact determination. Most often the dislocation of a disc occurs because of torn ligaments surrounding the vertebra in question. Such ligamentous tearing or weakening results in many forms of spine pathology producing chronic instability of the back. The reconstruction therapist is trained to locate ligament, tendon, and joint structural defects by palpation (touching) alone. Since ligaments and tendons are not readily seen on x-ray films, CAT scans, and MRI studies, palpation is an extremely valuable skill.

Mechanical Findings in Chronic Instability of the Back

In a 1959 published paper, George S. Hackett, M.D., F.A.C.S. pointed out the reason for chronic low back pain. He wrote:

> Chronic low back pain is caused more often by incompetent ligaments and tendons [unable] to maintain normal tensile strength than for any other reason. It is the cause of joint instability and is frequently confused with disc disability and arthritis.
>
> Pain has its origin when weakened ligament and tendon fibers stretch under normal tension and permit an abnormal tension-stimulation of the somatic [body] sensory nerves that will not stretch.
>
> The diagnosis is made by trigger point tenderness over specific articular ligaments. The diagnosis is invariably confirmed by intraligamentous tendonous needling with a local anesthetic solution which reproduces the local pain and sometimes specific referred pain with intensity, only to disappear within two minutes as anesthesia takes place.[1]

The chief of radiology at Northwest General Hospital in Milwaukee, Wisconsin, Thomas Roskos, D.O. affirmed Dr. Hackett's description and went on to describe the roentgenographic (X-ray) findings in chronic instability of the back. "Mechanical instability of back joints in general have limited ranges of motion, which comes from inadequate functioning of ligaments," said Dr. Roskos. "The joints and their ligaments will have sprains, excessive relaxation, tears, or some other injury. There will be secondary muscular splinting. Muscles attempt to take over the ligaments' function. In the majority of affected patients, there is a loss of normal lordotic curvature [inward curving] — the S-shaped curve of the spine in a normal upright-standing human being tends to straighten out. — especially in the cervical spine. There will be subluxation of the spinal facets, marked intervertebral foramina narrowing, serious disc space disruption — all coming from laxity, tearing, and loosening of the ligaments [see Figures 13 and 14]. This looseness produces more friction, more inflammation, and greater back pain in the neck. In the cervical spine, further mechanical changes include extreme limitation of hyperextension and flexion [the patient's bending ability] and a torticollis [an irresistible turning movement of the head that becomes more persistent, so that eventually the head is held continually to one side — known as 'wryneck'].

"On X-ray examination, as a roentgenologist, I'm really not able to visualize these boney changes until the patient's pathological biologic changes or soft tissue changes become well established. To see them on X-ray films, they have to be of long-standing so as to bring the hard tissue changes into view," said Dr. Roskos. "You should know that ligaments and tendons are not readily visualized on X-ray films. The secondary changes which occur in the cervical, thoracic, lumbar or sacral vertebrae are what's actually seen, and they give away that soft tissues holding together the vertebral joints — that is, the ligaments — are damaged.

"The same physiological malfunction from ligamentous pathology is found in the low back. Such malfunctioning is characteristic of the spine in the lumbar and sacral areas having mechanical instability," continued Dr. Roskos. "There is an anterior [front] or posterior [rear] slippage of one vertebral body on another. A kyphotic curvature [outward curving like humpback] — the opposite of lordosis — can come on

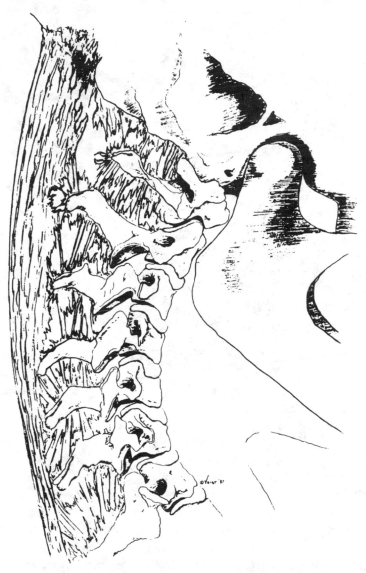

Figure 13. Torn and loosened ligaments in the neck created from chronic positional usage (as in typist, cashiers, and bookkeepers). It's work to hold up the head.

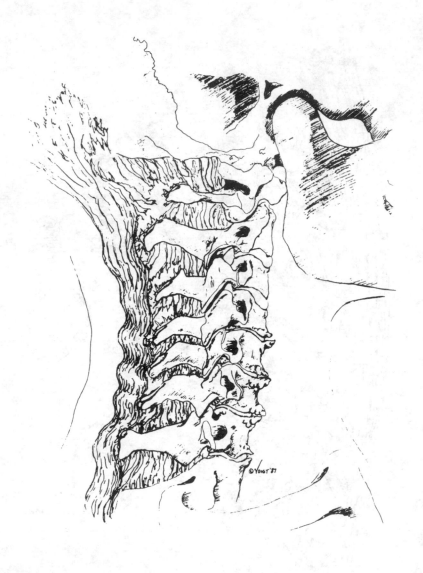

Figure 14. *Multiple levels of disc degeneration from overlax, torn, and loosened ligaments in the cervical spine resulting in loss of height, arthritic spurs, and disc disruption.*

[see Figure 15]. The patient may, over time, exhibit severe arthritic disease because of facette [or facet] jamming and arteriosclerosis [impaired blood flow]. This occurs as a result of the abnormal stresses placed on the apophyseal joints with erosion of the cartilage surfaces between them in the low back. The stresses produce osseous productive articular changes. Bones respond to stresses by making more bone in order to try and stabilize the joint. They attempt to fuse the spine into a stable position. The arthritis that's formed causes the neural foramena or 'windows' out of which the nerves exit to become narrowed. There will be impingement of the spinal nerves. Even a 2 percent narrowing can produce pain symptoms of this condition with spondylolisthesis."

Pathology and Reconstructive Treatment
of Spondylolisthesis

Forward or backward displacement of one vertebra over another, usually of the fifth lumbar over the sacrum or of the fourth lumbar vertebra over the fifth is called spondylolisthesis. This is a Greek word meaning "slipping away" or "falling free." It is caused by a lateral defect of the vertebral arch or erosion of the articular surfaces due to degenerative joint disease (DJD). Because of lack of ligamentous support around the vertebrae, spondylolisthesis causes backache radiating down the thigh and leg — a sciatica. The pain quite often disappears at rest but returns on exertion.

Reconstruction therapist Jack E. Smith, D.O. of Butler, Pennsylvania gives an excellent lecture on spondylolisthesis to budding trainees in the injection procedure which he advocates. Dr. Smith explains, "The most frequent encountered symptoms are generalized aching or low back discomfort which is aggravated by activity and eased by rest. Activities such as prolonged stooping, reaching, bending, working from ladders, descending stairs, walking down steep hills, lifting,

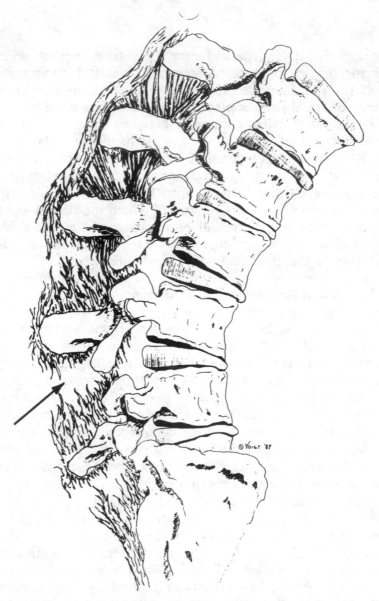

Figure 15. The low back with torn and weakened ligaments, thinning of the discs, and kyphotic curvature similar to what happens in osteoporotic "dowager's hump."

and other movements are examples. Sciatica may be present in 10 percent of the victims. The cauda equina [the bundle of spinal nerve roots below the first lumbar vertebra] may be stretched sufficiently to create motor weakness involving both lower extremities and occasionally sphincter disturbance [in the anus] with associated saddle sensory changes."

The cause of pain in spondylolisthesis is the postural adjustments; the lumbar lordosis (inward curvature of the spine at the lumbar region) converts the articular joints into weight-bearing structures. Osteoarthritic changes develop with stretching of the front and back longitudinal ligaments, the iliolumbar ligaments, the sacroiliac ligaments, and the lumbar muscle support. Nerve root irritation and compression set in.

The examining doctor may see a dimple in the back between the spinous processes at the spot where spondylolisthesis is taking place. His patient walks with a lumbar lordosis back or kind of swayback and flexion of the knees. X-rays readily confirm the diagnosis of spondylolisthesis and help to classify it into four degrees of severity. Osteopathic physicians and their medical doctor counterparts agree that 70 percent of patients with this condition have it at the fifth lumbar to first sacral vertebrae, 25 percent get it at the fourth lumbar level, and only five percent at higher levels. Most patients are told by orthopedists who have no skill in reconstructive therapy that they have a condition they must learn to live with or have fusion surgery. That is untrue! Reconstructive therapy permanently stabilizes spondylolisthesis so that there is never laxity of the ligaments, the initial cause of low back pain [see Figure 16].

Treatment involves injection of a tested proliferating agent such as dextrose with Lidocaine or PQU 1-4 Lidocaine, which is Dr. Smith's personal choice. For the sacroiliac and post interspinal ligaments he uses PQU 1-4 Lidocaine. Keep in mind that no less than 100 different proliferating agents are

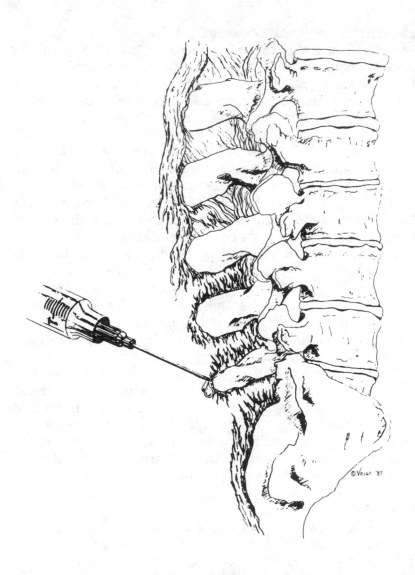

Figure 16. The low back with torn and weakened ligaments. Demonstrating the precise injection area at the fibro-osseous junction for reconstructive therapy.

employed for reconstructive therapy, and the one mentioned here is favored by just one of the reconstruction therapists. Dr. Smith may recommend the use of an ice pack for twenty minutes, if discomfort follows the treatment. He may also prescribe Darvon Compound 65™, Darvocet™, Tylenol™ plain, Tylenol™ number 3, Datril™ as needed. No hot tub baths are allowed for three days following the injection. Dr. Smith encourages light exercises such as walking and light stretching movements.

Causes of Chronic and Persistent Backache

Chronic and persistent backache with no obvious cause is one of the most common complaints of the human race. Yet, there is always a cause, and scientists knowledgeable in musculoskeletal disorders have designated five major groups or reasons for persistent backache. There are (1) chronic low back strain, (2) osteoarthritis of the lumbar articulations (spinal joints), (3) congenital anomalies of the lumbosacral region, (4) chronic inflammatory lesions of the lumbosacral joints, and (5) metabolic disturbances of the muscles, ligaments, tendons, and joints in the lower back.

Edward L. Compere, M.D., Professor and Chairman, Department of Orthopedic Surgery, Northwestern University Medical School, and William T. Kernahan, Jr., M.D., Attending in Orthopedic Surgery, Chicago Wesley Memorial Hospital, suggest that most people suffering from chronic fatigue syndrome characterized by persistent backache lead sedentary lives. They rarely participate in sports or even daily walks. "Many of these patients are working each day at tasks which they find uninteresting or onerous," say the two orthopedists. "Tired housewives, office workers and schoolteachers make up the largest numbers of the patients who are given the diagnosis of chronic back strain. They complain that they have no appetite, and they are tired all of the time. They appear listless, their tissues are flabby, and there is a lack of tonus in all of their muscles. Ligaments, which should be strong and taut in order to support the great load of the human body where the spine joins the pelvis, are relaxed and elongated."

Group five (5) needs to have the underlying pathology corrected before reconstruction can be successfully completed. Groups one (1), two (2), three (3), and four (4) respond most readily to having proliferants injected into their weakened, loosened, and torn ligamentous structures of the chronic low back disability.

You can see in Figure 17 that osteoarthritis of the lumbosacral spine may include the erosion of cartilage within the articular facet joints, spur formations about the margins of the articular facets, and the more obvious marginal osteophytes on the contiguous portions of vertebral bodies. Osteoarthritis results from the minimal traumas produced by everyday activities. As will be seen in the explanation of arthritis in Chapter Eight, marked osteoarthritic changes are more common in the spines of individuals who have worked at hard labor for many years. Any degree of instability of the articulations in the lower lumbar spine will increase the wear and tear on the articular facets and upon the margins of the vertebral bodies. Repeated overloading of the spine, as in lifting and carrying heavy loads, will result in reduced elasticity and efficiency of function of the intervertebral discs. Just as Dr. Roskos described, the disc space becomes narrowed and disrupted, resulting in increased motion between contiguous vertebrae, irritation of one vertebrae against the other, increased ranges of motion in the facet joints, and shifting of the weight back onto the articular facet joints. Wear and tear changes producing swelling of the ligaments, facet degeneration, and osteophyte (spur) formation will follow. Similar changes may occur from surgical removal of an intervertebral disc without

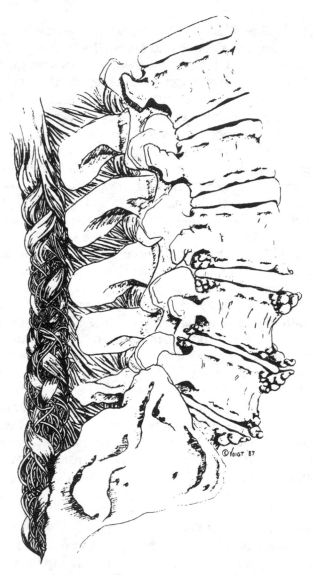

Figure 17. The low back with two degenerated, disrupted discs with resultant arthritic spurring stabilized by means of reconstruction of the ligaments.

fusing the spine. Fusion of spinal vertebrae results in hypermobility of the areas above and below the fusion.

As a person ages, ligament looseness brings on gradual disintegration and dehydration of intervertebral discs. Scoliosis or lateral curvature of the spine is usually associated with tilting of the fifth lumbar vertebral body toward one side. This tilt of the fifth lumbar vertebral segment results in an unequal distribution of weight on the articular facets. In turn, this leads to early degenerative arthritic changes in the overworked articular facet joints and may strike with severe persistent and chronic backache.

Likewise, chronic inflammation of the lumbosacral area may cause swelling and congestion in the subcutaneous fat, in the ligaments, and in the tendinous attachments of muscles to the sacrum and ilium. Chronic inflammation may be caused by focal infection, such as chronic tonsillitis, an abscessed tooth, gallbladder or urinary tract disease. Localization of the inflammation in the lower back is more likely to occur if the ligaments of the backbone are swollen from being stretched and overrelaxed as a result of, for instance, poor posture. Persistent passive congestion within any soft tissue structure will, within a short period, result in tenderness and aching. This is one of the more common causes of persistent backache. Also, rheumatoid arthritis and other low grade infections within the joints of the lower back may cause persistent low back pain. Reconstructive therapy can bring about unsurpassed improvement for all of these conditions.

Treatment Preferences of Injection Therapist Dr. Thomas Dorman

The newest procedure of choice in the musculoskeletal or orthopedic armamentarium is reconstructive therapy. Thomas Dorman, M.D. of San Luis Obispo, California, a reconstruction therapist, participated in a double-blind controlled clinical study that proved the value of this treatment (to be discussed in the next chapter). He states in a printed handout to his patients that most of the causes of chronic or persistent backache respond well to the injection procedure. Dr. Dorman declares, "It is possible with reconstructive therapy to stimulate ligaments to become stronger and shorter in cases where chronic pain is due to ligament relaxation."

Indeed, says Dr. Dorman, "In chronic low back pain cases when the doctor has made the diagnosis of ligamentous insufficiency, usually in association with a displacement of the sacrum or one of the lower lumbar vertebrae, the plan is first to ease the manipulative reduction with local anesthesia and perform the manipulation. Next, the ligaments are treated with a course of injections of a proliferant, usually for six weeks [see Figure 17]."

Dr. Dorman uses a mixture of three common substances that are altogether different from Dr. Smith's solution. These are:

(1) Dextrose, a type of sugar injected in concentrated form to produce a safe inflammatory response in the overly lax ligaments of the back. They are safe to use, assures Dr. Dorman, even in patients with diabetes, because the total amount injected is small. Dextrose has been used for certain kinds of nerve pain (trigeminal neuralgia) in which it abolishes the pain without upsetting the function of the nerves.

(2) Glycerine, found naturally in the body as a component of some fats, causes the injected tissues to swell temporarily and helps coagulate any blood that may pool in the tissues. It provides a framework or matrix on which new fibroblast cells can grow. The patient tends to notice some puffiness in the back at the injection sites after receiving the shots.

(3) Phenol, used in many injectable medications as a preservative because it prevents the growth of bacteria, induces the growth of new collagen connective tissue. It has been

used for many years in "face peels" by plastic surgeons since it is known to induce the growth of healthy collagen and elastic tissue thus removing wrinkles. It also has some properties of a long lasting anesthetic.

"These three ingredients have been used together since 1948 in Britain, where they were first introduced in the treatment of varicose veins," writes Dr. Dorman. "It is estimated that more than 100,000 injections have been administered throughout the body, though mostly for low back pain, without any permanent or serious reactions. The United States Food and Drug Administration has never officially approved or disapproved this mixture for use, but all of its constituents are approved." As pointed out here, FDA approval makes the use of such proliferants totally legal in the United States for use by any skilled and experienced physician.

Reconstructive Therapy for the Fastest Runner in Wisconsin

Something like the Dorman proliferating injection mixture was used to restore the running ability of a professional marathoner. Now age thirty-two, Marjorie McConnell (a pseudonym) of Madison, until her retirement from professional marathoning, was considered the fastest female runner in Wisconsin. She reached that pinnacle only through meeting and overcoming a host of physical obstacles involving her chronic and persistent backache. Marjorie, a speech pathologist, suffered with degenerative joint disease in her intervertebral discs. She went to the nearby medical center in 1985 because of her back pain, and was told by attending physicians that an operation was needed. "If you feel any worse," the doctors said, "we'll do surgery on your back. Let us know! Meantime, here is a prescription for Naprosyn™. Get the prescription filled and take this drug. We all have to live with pain. Oh, yes! You absolutely must give up running. Because it's bad for your back, don't do it anymore."

Even though she could not sit, stand, or walk without feeling excruciating pain in her back, Marjorie didn't like what she heard. Running meant everything to her. Then she happened to watch a television talk show (Channel 18 in Milwaukee) in which Dr. William Faber appeared as the guest. He spoke about his method of treating back pain with reconstructive therapy. Marjorie consulted him.

She proceeded to receive nutritional detoxification, improved bowel absorption, yeast (Candida albicans) elimination, and other aspects of biological therapy. It was after her body showed that it was free of toxic substances and infectious microorganisms that Dr. Faber gave his patient injections with a proliferating solution similar to the type used by Dr. Thomas Dorman. When her "before-and-after" examination results were reviewed, the marked improvement of her vertebral structure became obvious. She felt a great deal better, too, with almost no more pain after receiving only eight sets of weekly injections.

So, Marjorie took advantage of this improvment and ran in a demi-marathon (13 miles) against 200 of Wisconsin's best runners. She won! Then she traveled to Chicago to compete in that city's full-scale marathon and placed 37th out of 6,000 participants. Next Marjorie entered the ultra- marathon (50 kilometers or 33 miles) in Superior, Wisconsin and won. She became a nationally ranked marathoner and prepared for the 1988 Olympics. Qualifying times were given in events in Houston, where the 100-degree heat and 100 percent humidity hindered most of the marathoners. Marjorie McConnell was among those not qualifying. The Olympics went on without her.

She still runs but not professionally. In the summer of 1989, Marjorie gave birth to a baby girl. She ran with her bulging belly right through her eighth month of pregnancy. Marjorie reports that there never was any problem with her back throughout her pregnancy, labor, or delivery. When she was first telephoned for an updated interview about her therapeutic progress for inclusion here, she was out runing her usual daily eight miles.

Chapter Seven

Double-Blind Controlled Study Proving the Value of Reconstructive Therapy for Low-Back Pain

Can a proliferant, when injected into weakened or lax ligaments and tendons of the low back, produce an improvement in patients who have low back and sacroiliac pain? Are there any significant side effects or complications associated with reconstructive therapy when the injections are placed at points on and around bones of subluxated low back joints? These are just two of numerous questions posed by a research group at the Department of Rheumatology, Sansum Medical Clinic, located in Santa Barbara, California. Participating clinician researchers, including four medical doctors and a Ph.D., undertook a double-blind, placebo-controlled, randomized trial to prove or disprove reconstructive therapy's worth for the elimination of chronic low back pain. Their study was conducted throughout 1986, completed in March 1987, and published in the July 18, 1987 issue of *The Lancet*, the journal of the British Medical Association.[1] (Address reprint requests for this article to Robert G. Klein, M.D., Sansum Medical Clinic, 317 W. Pueblo, P.O. Drawer LL, Santa Barbara, California 93102.)

Despite the wide array of diagnostic tests and therapeutic modalities now available for low back pain, fewer than 28 percent of patients receive accurate explanations for their pain and even fewer receive satisfactory treatment. They usually take multiple medications but still feel constant low back pain. "You have to live with the pain," they are told by their doctors, or they are referred to psychiatrists after conventional treatment attempts (including surgery on the back) have failed. CAT scans, X-ray examinations, laboratory tests, and clinical studies of their musculoskeletal systems often appear normal or at most may indicate merely degenerative disease or so-called 'slipped discs.' X-rays, scans, and other tests simply do not show or in any way evaluate ligaments and tendons.

The Sansum Medical Research Foundation's F.D.A.-approved study of reconstructive therapy was conducted under the premise that there is a significant number of people with chronic low back pain who are suffering from torn or weakened ligaments and tendons. These ligaments allow for subluxation of the vertebrae in the sacroiliac region so that an "iliolumbar syndrome" sets in.

The Common Back Pain Factor:
Chronic Iliolumbar Syndrome

Described as a distinct low back pain syndrome (consisting of signs and symptoms that follow similar patterns) with typical findings of pain on one side of the low back, the iliolumbar syndrome can be produced by the hip flexion test.[2] There is also an exquisitely tender point at the rear portion of the iliac crest. The chronic form of this syndrome responds very poorly to the common methods of treatment of low back pain such as rest, analgesics, heat, and other forms of physical therapy. It is frequently aggravated by pelvic traction.

Whether or not the patient with iliolumbar syndrome (ILS) is treated, there are remissions and exacerbations of symptoms that may continue for a lifetime. Many patients complain of a constant ache that is aggravated by prolonged sitting and standing. The onset of this condition frequently follows a lifting accident or a fall.

Most likely the chronic ILS is the result of soft tissue injuries to the iliolumbar ligament and constitutes the most common form of low back sprain. However, sometimes it is found to be associated with radiculopathy (pathology in a nerve root that emerges from the spine). The condition of radiculopathy, which is disabling as well as painful, is usually the result of a recent or an old injury — most usually suffered in automobile accidents, otherwise in sports or from blows or falls. Less frequently, infections, growth disorders, or metabolic disorders may cause the nerve root inflammation. An example of radiculopathy is acute brachial radiculitis, which produces the shoulder girdle syndrome, evidenced by atrophy (wasting away) of the shoulder girdle muscles and accompanied by sudden onset of acute pain in the shoulder which may radiate to the arm or neck.

Some musculoskeletal specialists believe that most cases of backache originate from disrupted or degenerated discs. The clinical features of ILS have also been attributed to a facet syndrome in the lower back.

The best treatment for chronic iliolumbar syndrome is by infiltration of the iliolumbar ligament with proliferating agents — reconstructive therapy.[3] This is the treatment carried out by three medical doctors in the Department of Physical Medicine and Rehabilitation, College of Medicine, University of California, at Irvine, California. (Send reprint requests to Gerald G. Hirschberg, M.D., 6500 Fairmount Avenue, Suite 5, El Cerrito, California 94530.)

Drs. Naeim, Froetscher, and Hirschberg used the proliferating agent hypertonic dextrose as an outgrowth of the concept of musculoskeletal pain developed by Dr. George S. Hackett.[4] Their study involved sixteen patients with proven chronic iliolumbar syndrome, thirteen women and three men, ranging in age from 19 to 80 years old. The overall response was a significant recovery in ten patients out of sixteen.

Based on published research such as this, the Sansum Medical Clinic researchers believe that up to 50 percent of patients with nonspecific low back pain suffer from this iliolumbar syndrome. Damage to the ligaments of the low back is thought to come from loosening and stretching associated with normal pregnancy, major injury as from an automobile accident, or repeated microtrauma as from a physically stressful occupation. The Sansum researchers said, "These pain victims usually have an apparent leg-length discrepancy which is not a true anatomic inequality but rather is due to pelvic rotation or sacral torsion."

As a stimulus for their study, they accumulated a large body of case reports — about 250,000 patients — to support the use of reconstructive therapy for those with low back pain. From 80 percent to 92 percent of the patients having sacroiliac trouble from ILS seem to have been resolved of their conditions. Based on this anecdotal clinical evidence, the researchers undertook their double-blind controlled trial with proliferant solutions and placebo solutions.

What follows is, first, a summary of this study, its design, criteria for patient selection, procedures, and overall outcome. The Sansum Medical Research Foundation study is a convincing piece of science.

The Study

Combined with spinal manipulations, soft-tissue injections using the techniques of reconstructive therapy provided effective, conservative relief and, in some cases, permanent correction of chronic low back pain. Sansum Medical Clinic researchers found that a particular procedure of reconstructive therapy — developed thirty years ago in New Zealand — reduced pain and disability, without causing significant side effects.

The procedure, perfected from the work of American

George Stuart Hackett, M.D., F.A.C.S., by Milne J. Ongley, M.D. — then a New Zealand orthopedist and now a San Diego consultant in conditions of the musculoskeletal system — has been used by many physicians in New Zealand, England, Canada, and some European countries. Its chief exponents in the U.S., however, currently are among approximately 175 osteopathic physicians and a few medical doctors. The medical experts who are well-trained in reconstructive therapy are listed in the Appendix.

Sansum rheumatologist Robert G. Klein, M.D., says that the treatment is based on the theory that ligament damage causes many cases of low back pain. "Discs and joints degenerate when the ligaments no longer provide sufficient support," affirmed Dr. Klein in an interview.[5] "The manipulation moves the sacroiliac joint through a full range of motion, rupturing any microadhesions that may form in response to connective tissue immobilization, and corrects minor sacral malalignments.'

Then, Dr. Klein continued to say that the injection solution "induces inflammatory response that leads to fibroblastic hyperplasia [increased production and growth of normal cells] and the growth of collagen [a protein that is the principal constituent of white fibrous connective tissue as occurs in tendons and ligaments]." He conceded that this treatment approach triggers "a great deal of resistance from [traditionally practicing] orthopedists and neurosurgeons," but he noted as well that no one else has produced a double-blind study showing that any kind of conservative treatment works for back pain as well as reconstructive therapy.

Dr. Klein and his colleagues, Dr. Ongley, internist Thomas A. Dorman, M.D., orthopedic surgeon Bjorn C. Eek, M.D., and statistician Lawrence J. Hubert, Ph.D., randomized into experimental treatment and placebo groups eighty-one patients who had suffered low back pain for an average of ten years.

The experimental treatment group received vigorous spinal manipulation — intended to ensure a full range of motion — followed the next day by an injection of the three-chemical solution into specific fascial and ligamentous sites. A total of six weekly injections were administered, and regular daily flexion exercises were prescribed. The placebo group received sterile saline injections and less vigorous manipulation.

At three and six months after treatment, thirty-five of forty patients in the treatment group showed more than 50 percent improvement in disability scores, compared with sixteen of forty-one controls. Fifteen treated patients had zero disability at six months compared with only four on the placebo. And of twelve patients in each group who had pain radiating into the end of one or both legs, ten in the treatment group and two on placebo completely resolved at six months.

After more than twelve months, followup examinations were conducted. The patients who had received reconstructive therapy remained improved, and they have not required further treatments.

The People in the Study
The subjects for this back pain study were selected from groups of people willing to participate in a series of painful injections with only a 50 percent chance of receiving the real active ingredients. A mailing was made to a computer-generated list of 10,000 previously registered patients of the Sansum Medical Clinic. If a person had experienced back pain of more than one year in duration who failed to respond to previous conservative (nonsurgical) treatment, he or she might be the ideal candidate for the reconstructive therapy double-blind study. A total of 228 applications were returned by volunteers, and 117 patients were interviewed and examined, of whom 82 were accepted. All participants received full clinical evaluations, lumbar spine and pelvic x-ray ex-

aminations, laboratory tests, and other diagnostic procedures.

All of the 82 patients accepted for the study had previously undergone unsuccessful treatments. These treatments included chiropractic manipulation in 62 (76 percent), physical therapy in 47 (57 percent), massage in 40 (49 percent), inversion therapy in 20 (24 percent), acupuncture in 16 (20 percent), transcutaneous nerve stimulation in 10 (12 percent), corticosteroid facet injections in 10 (12 percent). One patient had gotten epidural steroids, one had experienced a facet rhizotomy (a surgical procedure in which selected nerve roots are cut at the point where they emerge from the spinal cord), and one had previously received injections of chymopapain (a protein-digesting enzyme derived from pineaple).

At the time of entry into the study 49 (60 percent) were regularly taking nonsteroidal pain medications for their chronic back pain, and six (7 percent) were taking codeine preparations. Patients were advised to stop all pain medications except acetaminophen (Tylenol™) and to avoid all other ancillary forms of treatment for back pain during the course of the trial.

Nearly all the patients (91 percent) reported that they were forced to change positions repeatedly after prolonged standing, sitting, or lying in one place. Seventy percent of them avoided lifting more than 30 pounds. Difficulty in rising from a chair was reported by 65 percent, and pain interfering with sleep affected another 65 percent. The participants also complained of inability to stand (59 percent) or sit (42 percent) for more than thirty minutes. Forty-eight percent said that they experienced constant back pain every moment, 32 percent reported difficulty with putting on socks or stockings, and another 32 percent had difficulty with bending or kneeling. Twenty-one percent were forced to discontinue or decrease their frequency of sexual activity because of back pain. Nine percent remained at home most of the time and an additional

4 percent stayed in bed most of the time.

Physical examination of these pain victims revealed that they had asymmetry of rotation and side flexion, presence of gluteal muscular irritation, but painless straight leg raise tests to at least 70 degrees. They were divided randomly by statistician Dr. Lawrence J. Hubert into the experimental or placebo group. Patients also were randomly assigned to one of the three treating physicians for the double-blind treatment and to a different treating physician the day of the manipulation, which of necessity was single-blinded.

A double-blind study or trial is the comparison of the outcome between two or more groups of patients that are deliberately subjected to different regimens. Those entering the trial are allocated to their respective groups by means of random numbers, and one such group (controls) receive no active treatment. Neither the patient nor the doctor is aware of which therapy is allocated to which patient. In a single-blind trial, the doctor usually knows what treatment — active or placebo — is being given to the patient.

The Sansum Medical Clinic Proliferant Injection Procedure

The experimental (proliferant) solution used in this study consisted of dextrose 25 percent (694 mosm/l), glycerine 25 percent (2720 mosm/l), phenol 2.5 percent (266 mosm/l), in pyrogen-free water to 100 percent. Because this solution may produce temporary irritation or burning sensation, it was diluted with an equal volume of 0.5 percent plain xylocaine (a local anesthetic frequently used by dentists) just prior to injection. Patients in the placebo group received sterile 0.9 percent saline. Each individual was administered six injections of approximately 20 ml of the same solution at weekly intervals. Each solution was identical in appearance and was prepared using sterile technique by a trained pharmacist. Phenol has a characteristic odor that might be detectable if a drop of solution were spilled. This potential source of bias was eliminated by adding phenol to the skin preparation throughout the study.

Patients in the experimental group were injected with xylocaine on the skin overlying the fifth lumbar spinous process. A three- or three-and-one-half-inch, 19-gauge needle was used for all injections. This rigid needle serves as a firm strut, thereby decreasing the possibility of an error in needle placement. All injections were made from this single insertion into the following structures: (1) tip of the spinous process of the fourth and fifth lumbar and associated supra and interspinous ligaments, (2) attachment of the ligamentum flavum along the borders of the fourth and fifth lumbar laminae, (3) the apophyseal joint capsules at the fourth and fifth lumbar and then the fifth lumbar to first sacral, (4) the attachment of the iliolumbar ligaments at the transverse processes of the fourth and fifth lumbar, (5) the attachment of the iliolumbar ligament and dorsolumbar fascia to the iliac crest, (6) attachments of the short and long fibers of the posterior sacroilic ligaments, and into the sacral and iliac attachments of the interosseous sacroiliac ligaments.

When the reconstructive therapists recognized a characteristic pattern of referred pain from the sacrospinous and sacrotuberous ligaments, additional injections were made from separate points into the sacrospinous and sacrotuberous ligament origins along the lateral sacral border. A maximum of 60 ml of 0.5 percent xylocaine was used in each patient of the experimental group. A patient in the placebo group received only 10 ml of xylocaine which was incorporated into 50 ml of normal saline so as to keep up with the same volume of solution and have the placebo take on the same appearance as the therapeutic solution.

Gluteal muscle irritation (of the buttocks), found to be a nearly universal phenomenon in chronic back pain, was treated in the experimental group of patients by an infiltration of 50 mg of triamcinolone (a corticosteroid) in 10 ml of 0.5 percent xylocaine. An injection into the fascial origin of the gluteus medius muscle was made with this anti-inflammatory agent. The placebo patients were injected with xylocaine alone.

A manipulation was then performed in the experimental group consisting of a typical sacroiliac lumbar roll.[6] The placebo group was given sham manipulation which produced no torsion across the lumbar spine or sacroiliac joints. Patients didn't know which procedure was being done to them because diazepam (an antianxiety agent) was first administered to them. The physician who performed the separate types of manipulations never gave the injections and never revealed who was in the placebo group or who was in the experimental treatment group.

Patients in the experimental group received the first of six weekly injections totaling 20 ml of proliferant. Approximately 85 percent of patients in both groups requested and were given premedication with intravenous diazepam, with or without demerol, to lessen discomfort. Each patient was monitored during the study for subjective complaints with a comprehensive questionnaire filled in during the week after each injection. All patients underwent complete blood counts, sedimentation rates, urinalyses, chemistry panels, and thyroid panels of tests. These tests were performed before initiating the study and after the fourth injection. Abnormal values were followed with repeated laboratory or clinical tests. No abnormalities of any serious nature showed themselves.

Assessment of the Study Outcome

The success of any treatment for low back pain must rest on the patient's subjective assessment of pain and disability.[7] Objective testing involving measurement of the subject's movement is "notoriously unreliable,"[8] and physical signs have been shown to be poor indicators of the pain and disability experienced by victims.[9] Clinical severity expressed by the patient is reported in the medical literature as not correlating with x-ray examination or CAT scans.[10, 1] For determining the extent of a participant's disability, the researchers at the Sansum Medical Clinic used a previously validated disability questionnaire designed by Dr. M. R. Roland.[12] There were thirty-three questions in all. The disability pain score was calculated by adding the number of positive responses. The questions emphasized loss of function in the performance of everyday activities rather than the individual's level of pain. Also, each patient marked a pain scale on each visit, represented by a straight line scored from a low of no pain to a high meaning severe pain. Disability and pain scores were assessed in a double blind fashion before the study's treatment, and then one, three, and six months following completion of treatment.

Each patient completed a pain diagram, which was analyzed for the area of pain by counting the number of grids marked at baseline compared to six months after completion of the treatment. The injecting physician was not involved in the evaluation process. All clinical signs were determined by an independent observer who had no other contact with the study patients. A variety of other clinical tests and examinations were performed, as well, to decide as to how the patient responded to the proliferant solution or to the placebo solution.

Breaking the Code and Recording the Study Results

At the study's conclusion, forty-one people were found to be in the placebo group and forty in the experimental group. One of the initial 82 participants had dropped out of the study. Overall, thirty-five of the forty experimental group of patients (87.5 percent) experienced a definite decrease in disability scores of more than 50 percent compared with sixteen among the forty-one patients of the placebo group (39.5 percent). Fifteen (37.5 percent) in the experimental group of patients had disability scores of zero at the conclusion of the double blind followup examinations compared to four (9.8 percent) in the placebo group. The pretreatment median disability score of the placebo and experimental groups were identical at ten. The six-month post-treatment median was seven in the placebo group and three in the experimental group.

The pain scores also showed statistically significant improvements at each followup visit. The experimental group experienced a much greater improvement. At the double blind evaluation six months after treatment, the placebo and experimental groups diverged sharply in their pain ratings. The patients receiving the placebo indicated over twice as much residual discomfort from their back pain as did the experimental group of patients.

The pain diagram grid analysis indicating areas of distribution of pain was not very different from one group to the other at the start of the study. Yet at the six-month followup, pain distribution reduced much more for the experimental treatment group than the placebo group. For example, twelve patients in the experimental and twelve in the placebo groups felt radiation of their pain into the ends of one or both legs at the onset of the study. At the study's conclusion, lower extremity pain had completely disappeared for ten of the twelve experimental group patients. Only two of the 12 placebo group patients showed any pain reduction in their limbs.

After six months of observation by the independent medical observer, his report was that side flexion and rotation asymmetry (not a healthy state) remained for just 45 percent of the experimental group but 54 percent of the placebo group. Irritation of the gluteal muscles of the buttocks remained for 58 percent of the experimental group of patients but 63 percent of the placebo group of patients.

In all cases, side effects of using the proliferating solutions were transient and mild. Patients in both groups complained of pain and stiffness for 12 to 48 hours after each injection. In no instance was this of sufficient severity to require bed rest or an absence from work. There was an increase in menstrual flow in two experimental group patients and in one placebo patient. Two experimental group patients developed postmenopausal spotting four weeks after initiation of treatment. One of the two women with postmenopausal bleeding had a dilatation and curettage and the other underwent a uterine aspiration with normal findings in both and no resumption of abnormal bleeding.

In only one case were side effects of sufficient severity to prompt withdrawal from the study. One of the patients in the placebo group withdrew after the first double-blind placebo injection due to a severe headache and cough the woman experienced, which resolved at a followup visit one week later. It is not likely that she had a reaction to the injected saline placebo solution.

There was not much difference in the laboratory values between the experimental and placebo groups. Most significant was that the light and electron microscopic specimens showed on biopsy a difference in the cellularity and collagen density between the untreated and treated ligamentous tissue. The treated tissue under light microscopy showed increased numbers of fibroblasts which were more sizeable and contained larger nuclei. These changes corelate with increased cellular activity and collagen production. The electronmicrographs showed denser collagen in the treated specimen that was biopsied.

Conclusions by the Reconstructive Therapy Investigators

The three physicians who treated participants in this study of reconstructive therapy, Drs. Robert Klein, Thomas Dorman, and Bjorn Eek, were trained in the medical mainstream of rheumatology, internal medicine, and orthopedics, respectively. Each was initially skeptical that the innovative approach suggested by Dr. Milne Ongley could be effective. After using his method in their private practices, they became convinced that reconstructive therapy was the most adaptive and precise procedure ever devised for chronic low back pain.

This rigorous testing proved that patients whose chronic low back pain had not been eliminated by conservative treatment will usually respond dramatically to the reconstructive injection regime. In reviewing the medical literature, it became apparent to the investigators that conservative methods of overcoming back pain had rarely been tested in such a manner.[13]

In contrast to prior results from conservative treatment, the reconstruction therapists found the following: "The experimental group showed statistically significant improvements in visual analogue and disability pain scores at one, three, and six months following completion of injections. These improvements persisted at followup three and six months after the 'code' was broken, without further therapeutic interventions. This was particularly impressive in that all usual medications and ancillary treatments were discontinued, and patients were encouraged to use their backs to perform previously painful activities. We were constrained by virtue of the study protocol from giving additional injections to residual areas of pain, although one would normally do this in clinical practice.

"Pain diagrams prior to and six months after treatment demonstrated significant improvements in the total area of painful tissue in the experimental vs. the placebo group," wrote the investigators.

They concluded, "In designing the protocol for this study, we were faced with the dilemma of testing each component of the system in order to isolate its relative contribution, or testing the system as a whole. We have seen dramatic clinical responses to each component of the system, and we have found that the long term high rate of success of this procedure requires that all the elements be included. Our concern was the necessity of having a large enough number of patients to be certain of adequate statistical power if the proliferant were the only variable tested. The repeated needling is painful, and it is a tribute to the study participants and a commentary on the desperate plight of patients with chronic pain that only one patient dropped out.

"The present study demonstrates a useful and safe method in the management of selected cases of chronic low back pain. The technique of treatment described and tested here is revolutionary and challenges many basic precepts. We believe these concepts and methods, once confirmed by others, will serve as the foundation of a new era in the succesful treatment of chronic back pain."

Reconstructive therapy is proven to help overcome persistent low back problems, but does it do away with other chronic joint pain troubles such as whiplash, migraine headaches, and other results of neck injuries? Does it do anything for degenerative arthritis symptoms, hurt knees, disabled wrists, injured elbows, dislocated shoulders, sprained ankles, TMJ syndrome, and malpositioned hips? Answers are "Yes," "Yes," "Yes," for all of these disabilities, and more.

In the chapters that follow you will learn how signs and symptoms are eliminated quite effectively for nearly every source of chronic joint pain on a regular basis by the trained and skilled physician's using reconstructive therapy techniques. Yet, "trained and skilled" are the keys to successful reconstruction treatment. Both authors declare that such training and skill should be verified by the patient before he or she takes reconstructive therapy.

Furthermore we state that all of the information provided here comes from physicians who utilize reconstructive therapy in practice, along with case histories supplied by them and their patients. This book is informational only and should not be considered as a substitute for consultation with a duly-licensed doctor. Any attempt to diagnose and treat illness or disability should come under the direction of your physician. To the best of the authors' knowledge and belief, all of the medicines, drug products, techniques, and other health care information referred to herein are legal. Neither of the authors have any interest, financial or otherwise, with any of the technique developers, product manufacturers, distributors, retailers, or other providers of any of the services, medicines, drugs or other items referred to herein.

The above few paragraphs should be taken as a disclaimer against loss or damage in the event the reader makes use of the information learned in this book. The practice of healing and medicine is both an art and a science. No guarantee is given or implied by this book.

Chapter Eight

Arthritis Symptoms Disappear with Joint Reconstruction

Arthritis is everybody's disease. If you live long enough, you will acquire some form of degenerative arthritis. Even if you do not suffer from acute pain or crippling, you'll experience various other joint symptoms such as limitation of motion, vague swelling, slight discomfort immediately prior to atmospheric changes, a feeling of warmth around the joint, skin redness, and other indications.

Medical historians exploring anthropological digs have found that joint degenerations with arthritis have always afflicted both man and animals. Evidence of degenerative joint changes is found even in dinosaur remains. Archeological findings going back 5,000 centuries show the disease affected primitive men and women.

Veteran reconstruction therapist Harold C. Walmer, D.O., F.A.O.A.S., D. M. A. of Elizabethtown, Pennsylvania, who currently is sixty-two years old, advised us that for many years he has been afflicted by symptoms of one of the degenerative arthritides. He told us, "I have osteoarthritis of my left knee, but I can work for over sixteen hours a day, being on my feet most of that time. I can also walk eighteen holes of golf and play a little basketball. Not being laid up with degenerative joint disease for me, is directly attributable to my receiving reconstructive therapy early in the onset of this arthritic condition. Here is what happened.

"In 1944, while playing football, I was 'blind-sided' by a hard-hitting tackle with resultant rupture of the medial collateral ligament of my affected knee. Not only did it sustain partial tearing of this ligament but the coronary ligament, as well. I had been a three- letter-winning athlete in college at that time, but the injury kept me out of sports thereafter.

"I saw many doctors to get relief for my knee but no effective treatment was prescribed other than diathermy. For several years I had what was then called a 'trick knee'. If I made the wrong internal twist, the cartilage moved and locked, and I was unable to straighten my leg," said Dr. Walmer. "This inability to extend the leg was always accompanied by severe pain and swelling. Back in those days surgery was not very successful for this type of injury, so I refused that particular treatment.

"Several years later I heard of reconstructive therapy (then called 'sclerotherapy' or 'prolotherapy' and then later 'proliferative therapy') and submitted to injection of my medial collateral ligament. The proliferating drug injected was Sylnosol which is no longer on the market. Within several hours of receiving that first injection series, I distinctly remember that my knee swelled and was very painful," advised Dr. Walmer. "However, when the swelling wore off in one week, the knee was much more stable. In fact, I went for several years without any knee trouble. Much later, arthroscopic X-rays confirmed that I had sustained a rupture of the medial meniscus. It is now 45 years since that original football injury, and, as I mentioned, I am quite active during work and recreation despite my having osteoarthritis and cartilage rupture. There's no doubt that my receiving reconstructive therapy then saved me from suffering with severe arthritic symptoms now.

"It was from this early experience that I became vitally interested in reconstructive therapy. I first learned of such a remarkably effective injection treatment while I was studying at the Philadelphia College of Osteopathic Medicine — more specifically in my anatomy dissection laboratory class with Earl Gedney, D.O. Dr. Gedney was the guiding light in the osteopathic profession, regarding reconstructive therapy. In anatomy classes, in 1949, Dr. Gedney taught my fellow osteopathic students and me how to inject the annulous [a circular opening or ring-shaped structure] of the lumbar discs. Later he lectured to the Eastern Academy of Osteopathic Medicine in New York City, as well," Dr. Walmer fondly recalled about his mentor. "He explained to us how, when a disc ruptured and lost height, a laxity occurred in the supporting ligaments with a resulting hypermobility. He explained how injection therapy administered to surrounding lax ligaments tightened the joint and prevented recurrent attacks of joint pain whether in the back, the knee, or anyplace else that the ligaments were torn, overly relaxed, or otherwise not functioning correctly."

Dr. Walmer added, "It has been my observation that various physicians — like myself — who finally evolve into being the best trained, the most highly skilled, and the most empathetic reconstruction therapists, are those who have been personally helped from receiving reconstructive therapy.

"I had another personal experience in the early 1960's that possibly led to a further touch of arthritis occurring in my low back. It also helped me to uncover a significant finding about supposed 'slipped discs'. At the time I was carrying fireplace logs into my home when I experienced a sudden, severe pain around my sacroiliac. I found myself unable to straighten up," continued Dr. Walmer, "and could only lay down sideways in the fetal position. The pain was severe, and I felt totally incapacitated. The pain radiated down the right leg and hurt like the blazes during any coughing and with all movement. My professional impression was that I had ruptured a disc.

When finally I could move, I went to a colleague and requested that he inject proliferating solution into my fifth lumbar facets and interspinous ligament. These were the connective tissues that I thought were involved with the pain. This injection procedure gave me absolutely no relief. The two spots I had selected were the wrong locations for the medication to work. I then requested that my right sacroiliac ligament be injected. This provided me with immediate relief of the pain.

"Although arthritis has lodged in this low back area and occasionally has me feeling some minor symptoms of weakness from time to time," he said, "the reconstructive therapy has again saved me from feeling the agony commonly associated with low back pain.

"There is a lesson to be learned from my experience. From clinical observations of hundreds of cases just like mine, now I know that many people with back trouble who are erroneously labeled as having a 'ruptured disc' are not the victims of that problem at all. In reality, these many so-called ruptured or 'slipped discs' are merely severe sacroiliac sprain of the surrounding ligaments. Serious orthopedic surgery isn't required as the corrective mechanism, inasmuch as reconstructive therapy does away with the low back pain and its beginning tendency toward one of the several forms of arthritis," concluded Dr. Walmer.

Forms of Arthritis Anywhere in the Body

The word "arthritis" whether diagnosed as present in the knee, back, shoulder, ankle, fingers, or anywhere else in the body always means the same thing. Literally, the term indicates the presence of inflammation of a joint (from the Greek, arth meaning "joint" and itis meaning "inflammation"). The combination word actually refers to more than 100 different joint diseases. Still, arthritis as most people know it consists mainly of two or three types — rheumatoid arthritis and osteoarthritis are most commonly recognized.

Traumatic arthritis comes from injury. Traumatic arthritis is the initial form that struck Dr. Walmer's knee; then it changed into osteoarthritis as time progressed. Traumatic arthritis comes from sudden, severe injury to a joint, usually from a fall or other accident. Osteoarthritis and traumatic arthritis are most effectively aided by adminstration of reconstructive therapy.

Rheumatoid arthritis responds less well because it is largely a metabolic disease relating to the lack of homeostasis in the body. Homeostasis is the physiological process by which the internal systems such as blood pressure, body temperature, or acid-base balance, are maintained despite variations in external conditions. Rheumatoid arthritis is a chronic condition that is usually progressive in nature. Its name signifies that it is somewhat similar to rheumatic fever in that both involve inflammation of the joints. The heart is affected in both cases — although to a greater extent in rheumatic fever. In rheumatoid arthritis several joints are involved, usually in a symmetrical pattern. For example, both hands may be affected or both knee joints.

The actual cause of rheumatoid arthritis is unknown although there is evidence that both physical and emotional stress tend to aggravate the onset of inflammation. Because of the physical factors, reconstructive therapy may be very useful as a relief mechanism for limitation of joint motion or excess joint play.

In contrast, osteoarthritis is a degenerating disease of the joints that results in fissures and cracks in articular cartilage. This form of arthritis almost always strikes only those in middle and later life. Its exact cause is unknown but previous trauma — either as sudden injury in an accident or as minor repetitive movements while working on an assembly line —

obesity, and age seem to be the major contributing factors. Just like rheumatoid arthritis, more women are commonly afflicted with osteoarthritis than men.

Usually coming on gradually without overt signs until the disease is well established, osteoarthritis affects the spine as well as other joints. Unless it involves the hip joint, the condition is not a crippling disease. That is because the body attempts its own healing by laying down calcium around the inflamed joint to splint its ligaments and tendons and restrict joint movement. In conventional medicine, the main treatment for arthritis is rest. The body attempts such rest of the part on its own by using calcium deposition as an agent of support. (See Figure 18, in which the damaged knee joint is splinted for stability and limitation of movement by the body's arthritic spurring with calcium. Also see Figure 19, in which arthritic spurring, bubble-like deposits of calcium, have formed on the cervical vertebrae in order to give support to the thinned and disrupted discs between these bones.)

Reconstructive therapy, administered not into the joint space but rather into the loose ligaments, can make the pain caused by osteoarthritis disappear. Injection with proliferants will not cause the calcium deposition to disappear, although one of the authors (Faber) wants to do a long term study on this subject. He believes the spurring will be shown to disappear if the joint becomes fully stable. Instead, these solutions merely strengthen the ligaments and tendons so that new fibrous cicatrix develops and the encompassing connective tissues resume their supportive functions.

Major Pennsylvania Health Insurance Company
Fails to Pay for Reconstructive Therapy

Today, osteoarthritis — the arthritis of wearing out and tearing down — degeneration of the joints — affects more than 36 million North Americans of all ages, but in particular

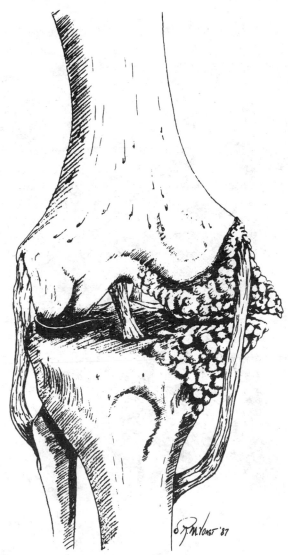

Figure 18. Damaged knee joint with loss of cartilage height, flaccidy of the ligaments, mechanical friction, and eventual arthritic spurring as the body's only self-applied means of stabilizing the joint.

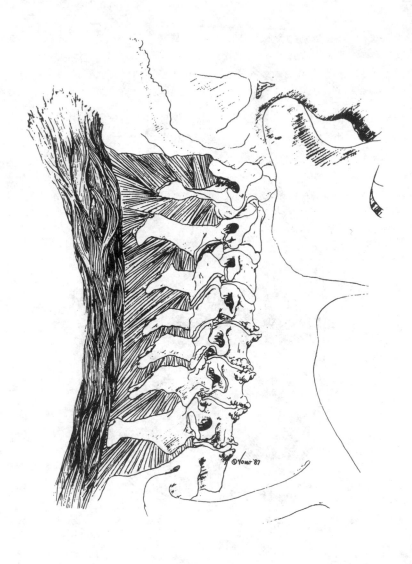

Figure 19. An arthritic neck having disrupted discs with new ligamentous growth from reconstructive therapy resulting in stabilization.

the elderly. According to The Arthritis Foundation, each year about one million Canadians, Mexicans, and Americans, all together, develop degenerative arthritis. Degenerative arthritis can occur in any joint, but the fingers, hips, knees, and spine are most commonly affected.

The Arthritis Foundation advises people that degenerative arthritis cannot be cured, but that is because this institution has not studied the beneficial effects of reconstructive therapy. If the Foundation had, it probably would be acknowledging by now that this exceedingly effective injection treatment absolutely eliminates the symptoms of degenerative arthritis and almost no other treatment is needed.

More than one public institutions has ignored the efficacy of reconstructive therapy. During our interviews, Dr. Harold Walmer provided us with one example of an insurance company that refuses to reimburse its subscribers for reconstructive therapy. Dr. Walmer was told by the major Pennsylvania health insurance carrier that if his study group of practicing joint reconstructionists could present supporting research to prove the efficacy of the injection treatment this health insurance institution would consider placing reconstruction therapy on its list of covered procedures.

"It was then that I collaborated with King Liu, Ph.D. and C. M. Tipton, Ph.D. to do a double-blind study on animal ligaments at the University of Iowa.[1] The credentials of Drs. Liu and Tipton were the finest of any researchers in the country regarding animal ligament research," said Dr. Walmer. "I instructed and assisted the research team in how to inject the animal ligaments with both sodium morrhuate and a placebo." For graphic illustrations of the effect of proliferants on animal ligaments, look back at Figures 3 and 4 that are reproduced in Chapter Four.

"Armed with this very supportive data, I scheduled a meeting with the prominent Pennsylvania health insurance carrier," continued Dr. Walmer. "At a luncheon prior to the meeting, the company's vice president, who at one time had been my student, told me to enjoy the lunch as it was all I would be getting from his insurance company. I replied to him that I personally wanted nothing from any health insurance company, as I was paid by my patients for treatment rendered. I explained to him that I was only acting in my patients' interest. I felt that the carrier's subscribers were paying a premium for a legitimate and proven treatment for which their insurance company was refusing reimbursement."

At the formal meeting, Dr. Walmer presented the case for reconstructive therapy reimbursement to the Pennsylvania insurance company's subscribers before a committee composed of physicians and consumer representatives. Across the nation, this doctor-run health insurance company has a system for analyzing new procedures by consulting with "specialists on procedures to evaluate for payment."

Unfortunately, the specialists called on for opinions about the efficacy of reconstructive therapy in this evaluation were neurologists and orthopedists, the two specialties in medicine most hostile to the procedure. Reconstructive therapy tends to eliminate the need for their services. Dr. Walmer was not privileged to see the specialists' reports immediately, but they were made available to him at a much later date.

"Some of the consultants claimed that they never had heard of reconstructive therapy, while others were in definite conflicts of interest inasmuch as the treatment effectively keeps patients with low back pain out of the hospital and away from surgery," Dr. Walmer assured us. "One of the radiologists claimed there were not enough human studies even though the procedure has been carried out since the 1920's. "Another doctor on the [evaluation] committee, [an internist] who had been one of my professors at the Philadelphia College of Osteopathic Medicine, criticized reconstructive therapy because he recalled a patient of Dr. Gedney's who received sclerotherapy [reconstructive therapy] and had to go to the Norristown Osteopathic Hospital for a shot of Demerol to relieve the pain following Dr. Gedney's joint reconstruction treatment." Dr. Walmer went on to comment, "Here we have a doctor who is an internal medicine specialist and is criticizing a procedure that he does not use for a condition that he does not treat. I explained to him that the standard alternative to reconstructive therapy — laminectomy — usually requires a postoperative narcotic and that today sophisticated reconstruction techniques rarely cause the patient to experience that type of pain.

"Other than myself, there were no other proponents of reconstructive therapy at the insurance company meeting. One influential member of the committee, the late Dr. Ray Solomon, who intended to speak in favor of reimbursement for reconstructive therapy did not attend. He claimed that he didn't know the meeting was to be held," said Dr. Walmer. "Dr. Jack Smith of Butler, Pennsylvania, a specialist in reconstructive therapy was on his way to attend, but the fog at Pittsburgh Airport prevented his plane from taking off. He never got to the meeting. The vote of this evaluation committee was nine to five against paying back patients for undergoing reconstructive therapy. Presently Workers' Compensation and various private insurance companies pay for the procedure, but not the individual State divisions [of this national health insurance carrier].

"Still, it's curious that the company pays for the hospital procedures of laminectomy and chymopapain injections [before chymopapain lost its therapeutic standing]. Both procedures command fees of from $1,500 to $2,500. Reconstructive therapy effectively treats conditions that both the above procedures treat but on an outpatient basis at less than half the cost. It is my impression that there are too few physicians practicing reconstructive therapy, and therefore we have too little political clout. Efficacy is not the issue," concluded Dr. Walmer.

Thus, this national health insurance carrier fails to reimburse its subscribers for a legitimate injection procedure that is less expensive, less painful, more permanent, and faster in rehabilitating chronic joint pain than any other treatment method.

Bones Respond to Stress by Making More Bone

Ellis V. Browning, M.D. of Yuma, Arizona was consulted early in 1982 by seventy-one-year-old Lorraine Victoria Magruder who suffered with generalized degenerative arthritis requiring her to wear special shoes for exceedingly sore and stiffened heels and ankles. Activity of osteoblasts (the bone-making cells in the body) for many years had deposited large amounts of arthritic bone spurs in the joints of her lower limbs. Mrs. Magruder had undergone considerable care from rheumatologists. Dr. Browning administered reconstructive therapy to Mrs. Magruder's feet, and her arthritic spurring and degeneration stopped hurting her altogether.

In July 1987, the woman consulted with Dr. Browning again. Her main complaint now was the development of severe shoulder pain radiating down both arms. The pains had not been relieved by her family physician, an orthopedist, a rheumatologist, nor by a neurologist. The two surgical specialists of course recommended different types of operations, of which Mrs. Magruder would accept none. However, the patient did take many injections of cortisone and many arthritis medicines. In fact, the patient had ingested so much cortisone that she displayed the iatrogenic disease, coracoid syndrome. This is a side effect of cortisone in which the shoulder bone begins to look like a crow's beak.

But the woman found relief at last by turning to

reconstructive therapy. Two injection series of proliferants administered by Dr. Browning to Mrs. Magruder's shoulder gave her complete freedom from her symptoms of arthritis discomfort. To this date (September 1989), the relief has remained permanent — no more arthritic symptoms of the shoulder.

By using this treatment, Dr. Browning was able to eliminate the symptoms of degenerative arthritis. How did he do that? The sodium morrhuate or any other type of the one hundred or more proliferating solutions that the doctor prefers, injected into the tendon or ligament surrounding the arthritic joint causes counter irritation. The new inflammation stimulates healing cells which we have referred to as fibroblasts. They travel to the torn or overly relaxed ligamentous tissue and lay down new fiber — additional ligament or tendon — and this causes the area to become permanently stronger. Strengthened soft tissues around the articulating bones provide greater stability and endurance to the joint. The main side effect, therefore, is less arthritis pain for the patient. The new fiber is a kind of protein material called "cicatrix." It acts as supportive binding material for the arthritic joint.

An unstable joint shakes around, causing friction and stress in the bones. Stress in the joint's bones brings on arthritis. A known medical law is that bones respond to stress by making more bone. Arthritis manifests itself by the deposition of too much bone with associated inflammation from the friction of instability. The arthritis has developed from the body's attempt to help itself, as we have mentioned before, by splinting the overly loose or torn ligaments. They have been failing to perform their appointed function of stabilizing the joint, so that the body must try and accomplish this itself with more bone.

For the patient the problem is that his or her joint then loses its mobility and roughens many times more than is tolerable. Pain results! Furthermore, the ligament remains torn or lax and the underlying problem does not get corrected. In contrast, when the ligaments and tendons are strengthened, the joint stabilizes and the arthritic process ceases.

For reasons related to the pathological process, arthritis medicines do nothing to cure arthritic symptoms. They merely mask them. Drug-oriented physicians are mostly treating the effects of joint instability — the inflammation — and not the known cause — the joint instability itself. Consequently, when a person receives reconstructive therapy all nonsteroidal anti-inflammatory drugs such as Advil™, corticosteroids which are anti-inflammatory such as Deltasone™, gold shots, and other standard arthritis drugs are discontinued.

In contrast, the doctor wants the body's response, inflammation, to the irritation set up by the proliferant to continue. Remember, the initial joint inflammation is not the cause of arthritis, rather it is a result of friction from excess movement between bones in an unstable joint. Excessive movement is not the cause of the problem but the result of the lax ligaments. A physician trained in reconstructive therapy introduces controlled inflammation by injection of the proliferating solution at precisely where it is needed to make the ligament or tendon permanently stronger.

Admittedly, discontinuing anti-inflammatory drugs appears to be in direct contradiction of present treatment regimens for arthritis. But with reconstructive therapy, benefits accrue from discontinuing the anti-inflammatory 'therapy'.

First Time Administration of Reconstruction Therapy Worked Well

Ronald J. Frankenheimer, age 72 and retired, was brought for medical help by his daughter to Robert Rowen, M.D., Medical Director of the Omni Medical Center in Anchorage, Alaska. Mr. Frankenheimer was suffering with the long-term complaint of osteoarthritis in the low back, a condition known as spondylitis. It was located between the third and fourth lumbar vertebrae. He also felt constant arthritic discomfort around the sacroiliac. He was practically bent over with pain when he arrived at Dr. Rowen's door, and this was his usual state of poor musculoskeletal health.

A recent magnetic resonance imaging (MRI) scan showed that the patient had degenerating discs at the level of the third and fourth lumbar vertebrae as well as the other vertebrae mentioned. He complained of chronic aching in his neck and his low back. Being told by orthopedic surgeons and neurological surgeons that nothing could be done until he was in bad enough shape for him to undergo a back operation, the misinformed fellow was actually waiting for his condition to get worse. Consequently, he was seeking no help and not even doing anything for himself. His daughter could not accept this kind of thinking, so she made an appointment with Dr. Rowen.

As it happened, the Anchorage physician had just returned from preceptorship training with this book's coauthor, Dr. Faber. Under professional supervision, he used different needling techniques, experienced the injection procedure himself, took care of patients, gave injections to them and to fellow students, and learned of the benefits and possible side effects of the various proliferating solutions.

"This was my first private patient in Alaska who required reconstructive therapy, for I rendered service to him only a few days after my preceptorship training with Dr. Faber," wrote Dr. Rowen in his report to us of this case. "I performed reconstructive therapy into his sacroiliac joints and into his lumbar spine. It was gratifying to give the treatment entirely on my own.

"Reconstructive therapy proved wonderfully successful for him and this made a firm believer out of me," said Dr. Rowen.

"Three days after my injection procedure, the man's daughter telephoned me reporting that her father was free of pain and absolutely joyful. She thanked me for giving aid to her dad so effectively. Then Mr. Frankenheimer got on the phone and said that he had awakened without pain in his low back for the first time in his memory. The patient was completely pain-free for the next four days. Then I saw him again, and no discomfort remained in his sacral or lumbar regions. He wanted more proliferating injections but not where it no longer hurt. Instead, he asked me to perform the treatment on his neck rather than repeat it for his back. I did so. This was the last time that I saw the patient, since he returned to Arizona," Dr. Rowan said.

According to an article in *Medical World News*, arthritis is the number one health problem of over 45 percent of Americans 65 years of age and older. *Forbes* magazine in its issue of February 24, 1986 estimated that back pain alone cost business $56 billion per year. Mainly because of arthritis, one out of four Americans enter nursing homes for their last years. History has shown us that this costs between $20,000 and $30,000 per patient per year, most of which is not covered by Medicare and Medicaid.

Dr. Rowan's experience with correcting Ronald J. Frankenheimer's sacral and lumbar arthritis and the arthritis of dozens of additional patients since, shows that this level of pain and its associated costs do not have to continue. Reconstructive therapy is a potential solution. It works for arthritis.

Chapter Nine
Neck Problem's Causing Whiplash and Migraines

While water skiing in the late spring of 1989, forty-nine-year-old Inez Sommers, a bank teller in Pell City, Alabama, underwent a critical fall in the water at a speed that exceeded thirty miles per hour. She rolled over four times as she scaled along the water's surface like a skipping stone. This severely injured Ms. Sommers' neck and right shoulder. She quickly developed excruciating pains and weakness of her neck, shoulder, arm, and hand.

The following morning, after experiencing a miserable night of pain and suffering, the woman was unable to hold a fork in her fingers or use her right arm. Any motion of her shoulder and neck brought on pain, and she felt muscular weakness in these areas. Ms. Sommers consulted a chiropractor for X-ray diagnosis and treatment, and in successive visits over three days he administered manipulative therapy. The patient did not feel any improvement whatsoever and became totally disabled. She found herself unable to count money at her bank teller's window or even perform simple household tasks at home. As it happened, Ms. Sommers had taken back her maiden name after a divorce, and she was the sole support of two teenage children, a dog, a cat, and a mortgaged house. When the teller did not perform her duties, there was no income.

After another four days of unrelenting pain and suffering, Ms. Sommers' disability was not getting any better, so she consulted a specialist in sports medicine for evaluation and treatment. More X-ray films revealed no fractures, and a simple diagnosis of multiple sprains of several muscles of the neck, upper back, and right shoulder with possible tearing and separation of the rhomboid muscles of the right side was made. The sports medicine physician also arrived at a secondary diagnosis of inflammation of the entire myofacial system of the right neck area, upper back, and shoulder. He prescribed medication against the pain, nonsteroid anti-inflammatory drugs, steroid injections, and daily physical therapy plus the application of a TENS unit for healing from electrical stimulation.

Two weeks of intensive physical therapy and medications failed to relieve her pain, muscle weakness, and disability. In fact, the patient's pains became more severe, and she could not raise her right arm any higher than six inches — even then with considerable effort. Combing her hair or feeding herself with her right hand was out of the question. Seeing this lack of progress, the sports medicine doctor re-evaluated the patient and recommended continuation of the therapy with the addition of special exercises for the muscles of her right upper back and shoulder.

For the next two weeks, the patient continued to deteriorate. She developed numbness and tingling in her right neck, shoulder and arm and suffered with awful pain radiating down the back of her right arm and into her fingers. She continued her physical therapy sessions faithfully without improvement. Ms. Sommers became quite depressed and felt desperate to get relief. She had not been working or receiving a paycheck for over five weeks.

It was then that Inez Sommers visited BioMed Associates, P.C. of Birmingham, Alabama, the medical clinic of Gus J. Prosch, M.D. Dr. Prosch, who had taken training and a preceptorship in reconstructive therapy with Dr. Faber, became her physician. The patient arrived for evaluation and treatment of her worsening disability. By now it was six weeks after the patient's injury.

Dr. Prosch's physical examination revealed, according to his clinical notes,"severe weakness in the entire right arm with serious limitation of motion in all directions at the right shoulder joint. Weakness of numerous muscles on the right side was determined and the most serious involvement was found in the deltoid, trapezious, sternocleidomastoid, supraspinatus, Infraspinatus, and rhomboid muscles. The pain in the right shoulder and arm is consistent with damage to the cervical spinal nerves of C4, C5, C6, C7, and the thoracic spinal nerves T1 through T7. Further examination of the inter-spinous and supraspinous ligaments in these areas shows that they are very relaxed and possess numerous areas of tender-ness to palpation."

In our interview, Dr. Prosch told us, "Because of the damaged ligaments, I recommended that the patient should have reconstructive therapy of the relaxed ligaments from the second cervical through the tenth thoracic vertebrae. And if the expected improvement resulted, other damaged ligaments could also be treated with reconstructive therapy. The patient agreed to receive the treatment, and I injected the supraspinous and interspinous ligaments of the entire cervical and thoracic spine. I explained to her that I wanted the in-jected area to become very sore for the following 24 to 48 hours, which would insure the best results. I advised her to apply cold packs on the day of injections and hot packs during the next two days. Proper nutrition and elimination was stressed to the patient as being necessary. She was ad-vised to return in two weeks."

Ms. Sommers developed good soreness the evening of the first injections and the following day. To Dr. Prosch's surprise, by the end of the second day, her pains in the right side of her neck, upper back, shoulder and arm totally disappeared.

She was able to move her right shoulder about 80 percent better. He thought that a few more sets of joint reconstruction injections would have been required for that kind of progress. Such fast resolution of the neck, shoulder, and arm pain was unexpected. The patient, of course, was delighted with the results from her first exposure to reconstructive therapy.

Unfortunately, after a week the previous pains from the woman's trauma began to gradually return, but not as severely as before the injections. During her second visit to Dr. Prosch she was given further reconstructive therapy. The solutions injected were strengthened by adding an additional cubic centimeter of sodium morrhuate. Ms. Sommers was advised by the physician to return for consultation in three weeks.

Following this second injection series, she was sore for about three days. Her discomfort then disappeared along with the associated muscular weakness. She felt quite comfortable and returned to work. Numbness and tingling had disappeared. Nearly two weeks more went by without pain or other symptoms and then, her problems began to come back again. But the pains and weakness were much less. Dr. Prosch gave Inez Sommers a third series of reconstructive injections and she remained free of pain for nearly three weeks more. Gradually the patient noticed that a much slower return of discomfort and muscle weakness came on. Each time she underwent reconstructive therapy, however, the pain stayed away longer.

Over time, her neck, shoulder, arm, and hand pains discontinued altogether. Presently (October 1989), Inez Sommers has been fully employed for the past two months and even though some pain returns from time to time, Dr. Prosch estimates that following another three applications of reconstructive therapy, especially to her cervical spine, she will be free of pain forever.

Anatomy of the Cervical Spine

The cervical spine is the most complicated articular system in your body. There are thirty-seven separate joints, and their function is to carry out the myriad movements of the head and neck in relation to the trunk and to subserve all specialized sense organs such as the eyes, ears, nose, and mouth. The seven small cervical vertebrae, with their ligamentous, capsular, tendonous, and muscular attachments, are poorly designed to protect their contents, compared to the skull above and the thorax below. The contents of this anatomic cylinder interposed between skull and thorax include carotid and vertebral arteries, the spinal cord and all of its front and rear nerve roots, and, in its uppermost portion, the brain stem.

The extremely flexible cervical spine balances a ten- to fifteen-pound ball, the head, on the outer masses (zygapophyseal joints) of the atlas. The head acts as a cantilever on top of the highly mobile neck. Normally, the neck moves over 600 times an hour, whether you are awake or asleep. No other part of the musculoskeletal system is in such constant motion. The cervical spine is subject to stress and strain in ordinary, everyday activities, such as speaking, gesturing, rising, sitting, walking, turning about, and even at rest, lying down. Normal function requires that all movment be made without damage to the spinal cord, the entire vascular supply to the head and neck, millions of nerve fibers passing through it, and the intervertebral foramina.

Is the cervical spine clinically important? Do accidents happen to it frequently? Very much so! In one epidemiologic study, over 10 percent of the population who were questioned by clinicians recalled having had at least three episodes of pain in the neck in the previous years.[1] Also reported was that, at any one specific time, as much as 12 percent of the adult female population and 9 percent of the adult male population experience pain in the neck with or without associated arm pain; 35 percent of people could recall such an episode.[2]

Another important clinical epidemiologic study of cervical pain disclosed that a history of stiff neck and arm pain was elicited in 80 percent of a population of male industrial and forest workers.[3] The same medical researchers conducting this last study, plus an additional colleague working with them did a second investigation which modified their findings. Together they found that 51 percent of 1,193 men in a broad spectrum of jobs suffered from neck pain. Of these workers, 5.4 percent of them lost time from work because of it.[4, 5]

There is an important relationship between backache and neck pain. During and after World War I, backache was seldom reported as a problem. No one seemed to have it. When World War II was well underway, backache was the diagnosis in 40 percent of patients admitted to a general military hospital with "arthritis and allied conditions." Most of the time their problem was in the cervical spine — the neck causing the back pain. The period between the two World Wars, therefore, saw backache from neck pain emerge as a major medical problem for the military, and for health care in general.

The expression, "Oh, my aching back," arose, but in the decade following the Second World War it was soon superseded by "Oh, my injured back." The notion of injury, at least to plaintiffs' attorneys, implies trauma, damage, and somebody or something at fault — culpability. This general concept of culpability emerged out of the coincidence of two events: (1) the introduction of workers' compensation programs and (2) more frequent auto accidents, especially rear-end collisions with resultant "whiplash." We will discuss whiplash injuries a little later in this chapter, but let us first look at compensating the worker for his job-related injury.

Workers' Compensation as a Source of Backache

In 1934, Drs. W. Jason Mixter and J. S. Barr attributed backache in nineteen patients to herniation of the central pulp portion between the vertebrae (nucleus pulposus). They demonstrated that cure could be achieved by means of a laminectomy operation, and named the condition "rupture of the intervertebral disc."[6]

At the same time that these "slipped discs" were being developed as a new musculoskeletal condition, all state legislatures and judiciaries in the United States were considering worker compensation statutes. The states passed laws that provided medical care and compensation for wages lost due to "personal injury that arises out of or during the course of employment and occurs by accident."

Lawyers think of "rupture" as a rip, tear, or bursting of a normal anatomical structure; thus, it was a "personal injury." Even in 1990, a worker with a backache who is given a diagnosis of "ruptured disc," may be compensated, irrespective of a defined discrete cause of his or her symptoms. Most important for the collection of cash is a surgical scar on the back. Indeed, for lawyers representing workers, the surgical scar suppresses arguments to the contrary much more reliably than the result of that surgical procedure.[7]

From 1934 to about 1955, orthopedic surgeons (who had newly emerged as specialists) and other clinicians, as well as lawyers and the courts erroneously believed that "ruptured disc" was the cause of most persistent and disabling backache, in general, and neck pain, in particular. These views changed gradually over the following decade, as the confidence of diagnosticians, the enthusiasm of surgeons, and the self-righteousness of the compensation bureaucracy faded and waned. Today, the cause of most regional backaches is not declared to be herniation or rupture of the discs. It's known, instead, to be laxity (sprain) of the ligaments — in many cases actual ligamentous tearing — so that joints wobble in a state of unsteadiness. Such wobbling gives rise to muscle spasm, nerve impingement, and strain of the surrounding soft tissue structures. Such stress gives rise to pain along the spine.

Backaches are admittedly indeterminate. Documented slipping of the disc is rather commonly found in people who have no pain or other problems with their backs.[8] "Backache" is no longer a surgical disease. Greater than 80 percent of such patients may be expected to get well on their own or feel much better in two weeks, with most of the remainder recovering as the result of their receiving reconstructive therapy. Of course, the majority of physcians are not yet cognizant of reconstructive therapy so that much of the time the 20 percent of patients who don't have spontaneous resolution of their backaches just linger in discomfort for unlimited periods of time while they shuttle from doctor to doctor.

Certain symptoms occur in those people who experience minor and/or major trauma of the neck. These traumas occur most likely because of the anatomical difference between the cervical vertebrae and all of the other vertebrae in the spine.

Diagnosing Common Complaints in the Cervical Spine

The most common complaints sustained by people who have injuries of the cervical spine are pain and paresthesia (spontaneously occurring abnormal tingling sensation — feelings like pins and needles). The most common words used by patients to describe nerve root (radicular) symptoms in the neck are "electric," "shock-like," "radiating from the beginning of the cervical spine to its distal end," "traveling," "a narrow band," "bright," "sharp," "lancinating," and definitely "intermittent." Words used to describe pain arising from the deepest neck structures are "boring," "aching," "deep," "severe," "continuous," "not traveling," "in a very large vague area," "difficult to localize," and "more at the top than the bottom or distal."

Far more commony involved are such structures as ligament, tendon, capsule, anulus (ring-shaped structure in the fibrous sheath), muscle, and surrounding tissue attached to these structures. Pain syndromes in the cervical spine tend to be intermittent and episodic. There is no correlation between clinical symptoms and signs and possible findings on x-ray films. Diagnostic x-rays hardly show any cervical spine pathology at all when pain relates to the neck.

The chronic cervical syndrome is characterized by superficial pain in various parts of the head, face, ear, throat, or sinuses, as well as sensory disturbances in the pharynx, dizziness, tinnitus with diminished hearing, and blurred vision or pupillary changes. Certain vasomotor disturbances are also included with neck pain such as sweating, flushing, lacrimation (tearing), and salivation. All these are related to the anatomical arrangement of the sympathetic nervous system in the cervical spine. In addition, there may be headache, nystagmus (rapid involuntary movements of the eyes that may be from side to side, up and down, or rotatory), nausea, vomiting, and suboccipital tenderness (soreness under the saucer-shaped bone of the skull that forms the back and base of the cranium).

In impaired cervical spines, 30-45 degrees of rotation of this area will kink the neck arteries. Add in osteoarthritis, disc disorders, and facet disease, and you have vertebral artery compression that can produce serious symptoms of degenerative disease. An immediate effect of impairment of the neck arteries is that it will cause a person to faint.

Issues in Treating the Cervical Spine

A main rule followed by clinicians who are informed about the musculoskeletal system is to avoid the use of drugs for their patients or to use them sparingly and temporarily, as primary methods of management in cervical spine disorders. Unfortunately, training in medical school on the musculoskeletal system is so inadequate that drug treatment is the usual therapeutic approach taken when the doctors get out into practice. Also, many unnecessary operations on the cervical spine are being done. Of a total population of patients seeking relief from pain in the neck or head, John H. Bland, M.D., Professor of Medicine-Rheumatology, the Rheumatology and Clinical Immunology Unit, University of Vermont College of Medicine at Burlington, says that only 1 percent require surgery. He adds that there is no correlation between available range of motion and disability. And the doctor should not recommend an operation merely on the basis of x-ray findings, abnormal CAT scans, and MRI findings.[9]

The most common issues in cervical spine practice are those of pain, its localization, and the identification of the structure that is the origin of the pain. If the pain-sensitive structure is not known, there is no point in proceeding to give therapy, says Dr. Bland. Traditional techniques of clinical investigation using x-ray, myelography, CAT scans, and other diagnostic methods do not reveal sources of pain. The patient knows subjectively, and the doctor with educated fingers can palpitate the spine and predict places that hurt. The spine usually feels mushy in certain spots, and pain will be reported by the patient when those spots are pressed. These are morphological changes in the structure that are the best indications of pathology being present. The most effective doctor is the one who identifies the pain-sensitive structures and then judiciously applies reconstructive therapy.

Meanwhile, a startling truth has arisen. Did you know that neck injuries from wearing seat belts are becoming more common? This is the significant question asked by Thomas A. Dorman, M.D. of San Luis Obispo, California in his September 1989 Practice Newsletters for patients. Dr. Dorman writes:

"Now that we restrain ourselves with seat belts, with front end collisions the head is tossed forwards and backwards uncontrollably." He describes the result as "whiplash." You will remember Dr. Dorman as one of the team of four physicians who performed the placebo-controlled, double blind study on reconstructive therapy that we discussed at length in Chapter Seven.

Dr. Dorman continues, "Imagine a heavy object, a head, attached by strings serially to a row of blocks, the vertebrae. The strings in this analogy are ligaments. Next, in your imagination, whip the head forcefuly back and forth. If an injury is done would you not expect it in the strings? It would seem that ligaments are at risk in whiplash injuries. Though there has been some doubt in the past, it is now known that ligaments are indeed injured and are a source of pain." Whiplash injuries do produce much pain.

L. Terry Chappell, M.D. Corrects a Whiplash Injury

Alfred Porman of Bowling Green, Ohio, a 36-year-old factory worker, was driving to work at around 60 miles an hour when another car stopped short in front of him, and he sharply struck its rear end. The collison caused his head to smash against the windshield, and he suffered a violent whiplash injury to his neck. The auto impact was so great that he was thrown out of his chest restraint and his head broke off the rear view mirror. Subsequently, Al Porman suffered from severe headaches, burning and numbness in the back of his head, dizziness, nausea, and pain in his eyes. He was unable to sleep at night because of the pain. The agony of his neck and head awakened him, kept him prowling the house during the morning's wee hours. Needless to say, he was quite irritable in the daytime.

Alfred tried to work, but his factory job required a great deal of lifting, which he found extremely painful. He also tried to keep up with another, part-time farm job, but the extra work became almost impossible to sustain. Survival for him between bouts of pain consisted of visits to an extraordinarily skilled chiropractor, Dr. Neil Aldredge of Findlay, Ohio, who would adjust him frequently. The adjustments helped for a day or two, but unfortunately, they did not last, and Alfred's vertebrae quickly slipped out of place again.

Upon referral by Dr. Aldredge, the patient visited L. Terry Chappell, M.D., medical director of the Celebration of Health Center of Bluffton, Ohio, for an evaluation of his condition. Dr. Chappel, another one of Dr. Faber's reconstruction therapy preceptors, reviewed Alfred's x-ray films, did a thermographic study on him, examined him physically, and performed a clinical analysis. Thermography, a technique for measuring and recording the heat produced by different parts of the body, by using photographic film sensitive to infrared radiation, proved invaluable. These thermograms, produced and interpreted by Philip Hoekstra, Ph.D., President of Thermoscan, Inc. of St. Clair Shores, Michigan, showed that Alfred had severe inflammatory processes in six different muscles on the right side of his neck and upper back. The muscles were in spasm because the ligaments of the cervical spine were loose and not holding his vertebrae in place.

Dr. Chappell recommended a course of reconstructive therapy which he administered. The patient's chiropractor continued to adjust him prior to each session. By the end of the third injection treatment, Alfred felt much improved. His migraine-type headaches had disappeared. Eyes stopped hurting, and his muscles in the neck and along one shoulder remained only slightly stiff instead of in severe spasms all the time. He completed his course of six injection sessions. At their conclusion, Alfred Porman had no more symptoms of discomfort whatsoever.

Dr. Chappell decided to wait another two months before

he repeated the thermography test to see if the treatment was holding as well as it appeared to be doing clinically. The repeat thermograms did show dramatic improvement in Alfred's neck, back, head, and shoulder. The inflammation was gone. He is now back working vigorously at his two jobs and has no complaints.

The Nature of Whiplash

Whiplash injuries arise from force being placed against the soft tissues of a person's occipitocervical area (in the spine at the back of the head and neck) as occurs in the sudden stop during a collison from the front or rear in an automobile accident. The soft tissues involved in the pain process mostly are ligaments and tendons. Nerves are damaged as well and bring on sharp pain from injury of the fibrous ligamentous bands through which they run. Contraction and expansion of blood vessels that rupture cause an increased content of blood in the traumatized area and fluid swelling. Often, both internal bleeding and swelling complicate the pain picture and produce more disability. The large neck muscles go into spasm, too.

Because a disc may be compressed and have less height, a whiplash victim will experience more vibration and tension on the ligaments binding together the neck and midback bones. The injured person's entire bony structure in the spine tends to become unstable. The muscles kick in and try to splint the back joints in place. Eventually the muscles go into rigid spasm by attempting to fill a supporting function like bone rather than a mobility function as they are supposed to do. Additionally, friction created by the disc herniation with associated squashing of the cartilagenous intervertebral material cause bulging, so further rupture takes place.

"The traumatic force of a rear-end collision exhausts itself in injury to the soft-tissue structures, without skeletal lesions, hence presenting no X-ray evidence of trauma. In the scale of pain sensitivity, periosteum ranks first, followed by ligaments, fibrous capsular structures, tendons, fascia, and finally muscle," write five physician reconstruction therapists.[10] They explained that collagenous perforating fibers, known as Sharpey's fibers, run perpendicular to the bony surface of the neck vertebrae. Tensile strength is diminished where the collagenous fibers separate to enter the "pores" of bone, and this is where injury is most frequent in whiplash. The symptom of pain occurs when normal tension on an injured ligament stretches the relaxed ligament fibers, resulting in abnormal stimulation of the sensory nerves because the nerve fibers do not stretch.

When normal healing occurs, bone and fibrous tissue proliferate at the fibro-osseous junction that Dr. George S. Hackett described in his more than half-a-dozen clinical journal articles and definitive book monograph on the subject of reconstructive therapy. We have given references for these publications throughout this text.

As we said earlier, the back of the head and neck are more susceptible to injury than any other part of the spine because of this anatomic region's great mobility. Also, the head is a larger object resting on the spine, which provides a much smaller base. The stretching, tearing, bleeding, and organization of clots which follow such an injury cause the ligaments to lose their normal resiliency and strength. They go into a state of chronic relaxation which predisposes the joint to further injury and causes friction into joints. The result is joint pain in the neck.

Whiplash is a Pain in the Neck to Society too

Daniel O. Kayfetz, M.D. of Pittsburg, California, an orthopedic surgeon and medical expert witness in whiplash injuries, wrote in the *Medical Trial Technique* Quarterly (for lawyers):

As more horses leave the nation's highways, and are put, instead, under automobile hoods, the problem of the so-called "whiplash injury to the neck" becomes a greater headache, both literally and figuratively. The term "whiplash injury" is, admittedly, a poor one. It describes, perhaps inadequately, a mechanism of trauma, like the old terms "bumper fracture" and "side-swipe fracture," rather than a specific pathological (changes in tissue due to disease or trauma) entity, which would be more desirable. The injured structures in the neck are generally confined to the soft tissues, among which ligament (a band of flexible, tough, dense white fibrous connective tissue) to bone and mus-culotendinous (pertaining to both muscle and tendon, the latter a band of dense fibrous tissue forming the ter-mination of a muscle and attaching the latter to a bone) attachment to bone rank as the more frequent causes of prolonged disability.[11]

Injuries due to whiplash-like motions have become a pain in the neck not only to their recipients but also to society at large. They have become a source of income for attorneys and the entire court system. A convenient dumping ground to which many whiplashed patients have been relegated is the so-called "legal-suit-happy group." Cures are presumably achieved in this group by attorneys administering "cash transfusions" to injured plaintiffs.

Writing in the September 15, 1989 issue of *Hospital Practice*, John G. Curd, M.D., Head of the Division of Rheumatology at Scripps Clinic and Research Foundation in La Jolla, California, and Roger P. Thorne, M.D., Head of the Section of Spinal Surgery at the same institution, describe how whiplash and allied back disorders affect to society. They write:

Still another poor candidate for [back] surgery is the

143

patient in the midst of litigation or with pending workmen's compensation. It sometimes happens that the settlement miraculously effects a cure. In the absence of classic indications, we advise delaying any decision to operate until the legal case is over, if only because surgery inevitably raises the stakes and prolongs the litigation.[12]

However, hope is in the offering, for it has been observed for almost forty years that reconstructive therapy does away with whiplash injury, an announcement which now will be welcomed by auto accident defendants and their attorneys.

Reconstructive therapy is the treatment of choice for patients bothered by pain and associated annoying symptoms a month or more after sustaining occipitocervical injuries. Reconstructive therapy, as has been described, stimulates the production of new fibrous tissue and bone cells at the site of predilection of such injures, the fibro-osseous junction. The strengthening of this injection area occurs over a period of six to eight weeks following the intraligamentous injection against bone of proliferant solutions.

Dr. Kayfetz rendered reconstructive therapies to 189 patients, seen over a five-year period. Treated by this method, 79 percent of these people were injured in automobile accidents. In 81 percent the injuries included other areas in addition to whiplash sites. Fifty-five percent had felt their pain and concomitant symptoms for more than three months and 21 percent for over a year. Yet, this orthopedic surgeon who is skilled in reconstructive therapy corrected 60 percent of them with "excellent" results. Also he got "good" results in 8 percent, "fair" results in 18 percent, and "poor" responses in only 14 percent.

An "excellent" result was considered achieved when there were no residual symptoms left; "good" meant there was no pain in the neck, head, or upper extremities, but some residual limitation of motion or other mild nondisabling symptoms, "fair" consisted of occasional pain in neck, head, and upper extremities, and associated mild nondisabling symptoms, and a "poor" response was judged to have occurred when there was no relief of pain. All of the "excellent," "good," and "fair" results totaled 86 percent of Dr. Kayfetz's patients. These patients themselves considered their results to be satisfactory.

As it happens, injury to the cervical spine of the patients described by Dr. Kayfetz frequently resulted in headaches for the traumatized victim. Headache is commonly associated with occipitocervical (whiplash) injuries.

Migraine Headaches from Cervical Spine Injury

Recurrent, severe, and unmitigating migraine headaches may arise from injuries to the cervical vertebrae. Migraine is a term that comes from French and whose literal meaning is half cranium. Migraine has that name because the pain usually affects only one side of the head and typically is preceded by an aura. The migrainous aura usually affects the patient's eyesight with brilliant flickering lights or blurring of vision. Of course, it also may be traced to such disorders as high blood pressure, atherosclerosis, intercranial aneurysm, allergic reaction, some subtle glandular abnormality, and emotional stress or chronic anxiety. A neurotic perfectionism is one of the personality traits that many migraine sufferers have in common.

When known trauma is pinpointed as the responsible factor, migraine headaches may be permanently correctable using reconstructive therapy. This was the case for fifty-one-year-old Marilyn A. Fischer of Harrisburg, Pennsylvania who was the debilitated victim of migraines for forty years.

"I started having headaches at age eleven, after I was hit by a car while I was crossing the street," explained Mrs. Fischer. "My hospitalization lasted four months and rehabilita-

145

tion went on for another eight months. I had sustained a broken neck with five crushed cervical vertebrae. The migraine headaches began in earnest near the end of my rehabilitation period. At first treatment for them was given to me in the form of pain pills. The pain-killers got stronger and stronger until finally when I was twenty-five years old and able to make sense out of my life, I realized that I was a drug addict. My dependency on prescriptions was no better than the dope fiends who feed their illegal habits with street drugs.

"I began going to different doctors then, looking for some therapy — a laying on of hands, medicines, herbs, prayer, hypnosis, traction, massage, biofeedback, manipulation, injections, some wonder drug — anything to relieve my pain without narcotics, psychotropics, or other pills that altered one's ability to think. I must have tried several dozen therapies and a like number of doctors," said Mrs. Fischer. "However, my pain continued without letup. It affected my marriage and eventually I did get divorced. It affected my job and even the labor union was unable to keep me from getting fired. At other factories at least once a week in the middle of the day, I'd have to leave my work as a quality-control inspector on an assembly line to go home. There I would lower my house shades, crawl into bed, pull the covers over, and wait for the pain to pass."

Mrs. Fischer explained, "Mine was a sick headache accompanied by nausea, quesiness, and vomiting. The aura that preceded it was visual — flashes of light in the center of my vision or flickering sensations in one eye. I felt apprehension, irritable, and restless whenever I suspected an impending attack. I felt sensitivity to light, sweating, and disorientation. The headaches varied in frequency, occurring every day or only sporadically, sometimes hitting hard just before my menstruation. Other times I would awaken from a restless sleep with a migraine."

Life improved markedly for the patient when she tried one more technique administerd by Dr. Harold C. Walmer. Dr. Walmer, as he does with most patients who suffer with whiplash, migraine, and other musculo-skeletal symptoms resulting from occipitocervical injuries, offered this woman reconstructive therapy. The injection technique works for whiplash, migraine, and other head and neck problems no matter how old the neck injury.

In nine weekly treatments, Mrs. Fischer got rid of migraine headaches that had been a forty-year part of her life. "I had prayed," she said. "I prayed, 'Dear Lord, you just have to help me get over this pain. You don't want me to suffer this way, and I know you're going to fix it.' And He did. He sent me to Dr. Walmer with reconstructive therapy. I haven't felt that awful migraine for over four years. I think that I am cured!"

At this writing, Marilyn Fischer has remained without headaches of any kind.

Recognizing Cluster, Migraine, and Tension Headaches

Writing in *Postgraduate Medicine*, Lester S. Blumenthal, M.D. of La Jolla, California states that experience of the individual physician indicates to him or her which are the different forms of cluster, migraine, and other types of tension headache, as well as postconcussion and whiplash headache, that are consequences of traumatic cervical spine injury.[13] He suggests a means of recognizing the migraine or other form of headache that comes from whiplash.

Dr. Blumenthal says that physical examination of a person who has some form of chronic headache and has sustained an injury to his cervical spine may reveal some characteristics that relate to the injury. The injured individual carries one shoulder lower than the other and holds the head rigid. There is a limitation in the range of active and passive motion of the head on the neck, sometimes in all directions. Pain is probably present. Compression of the head downward on the neck often increases the pain. Manual traction of the head upward from the neck may relieve it. Pain may also be increased by isometric pressure at the back of the head, whereas pressure at the curve of the neck may decrease it.

Muscle spasm of one or more of the supporting rear neck muscles will probably be apparent. There will be small, tender areas of spasms in other muscles that might be considered trigger points. Changes in neurological reflexes will have taken place. And with acute injury, there might be loss or reversal of the normal lordotic curve or increased laxity of supporting ligaments, or both. The range of motion is so restricted — either by spontaneous spasm, by attempting to hold the head rigidly on the neck, or by prolonged use of a cervical collar — that a cycle of muscle spasm, reflex pain, weakness, and atrophy of the soft tissues is set up.

The best treatment for headaches other than those caused by some metabolic or biological cause is reconstructive therapy. This is true because the injection procedure accomplishes most of the clinician's therapeutic goals: (1) removal of the tender trigger areas which serve as foci of the injured person's referred pain and spasm, (2) correction of malalignments, subluxations, and restricted range of motion to as near normal as possible for that individual, and finally (3) strengthening of the local supporting ligaments and tendons to prevent further malalignment and subluxation. Achieving these aims, migraines will disappear for the patient.

Harish P. Porecha, M.D. of Modesto, California, trained in a preceptorship by Dr. Faber, accomplished these goals for his chronic migraine headache patient, Audrey Connestoga, a telephone operator, age forty-two and unmarried. The headaches truly interferred with her ability to work. Her fellow operators joked that it was the continuous voice sounds in her ears that brought her pain like sledgehammers, but

Audrey could trace her problem to 1981 when she hurt herself skydiving.

Dr. Porecha described his patient's symptoms and treatment to us in late September of 1989. "She had severe migraine headaches requiring Demerol™ and Vistaril™ shots," he wrote. "She had several neurological tests done, all of which were negative. She had normal reflexes in the neck. The latest treatment that my patient received was in May 1989 when I administered [reconstructive] injection therapy with Discus™ 2.2 cc, sodium morrhuate 1/2 cc., lidocaine 2.2 cc. The reconstruction therapy was given [to the patient] from the seventh cervical to the occiput, and she was also on treatment with Prozac™ for antidepression.

"She improved so much that she started to enjoy living once and again. She even resumed her sport/hobby — sky diving with a parachute — jumping out of an airplane at 15,000 feet," said Dr. Porecha. "She certainly became a more lively person. I administered another series of injections to her neck about three months after the first set and she has been continuing to improve with almost no headache medication necessary.

"It was quite gratifying to see this woman do so well with elimination of her migraines. She was extremely grateful for the excellent therapy being available for her neck area," Dr. Porecha concluded.

Nontraumatic Neck Pain Resolved
with Joint Reconstruction

Another report we received about neck pain resolved with reconstructive therapy came from Dietrich K. Klinghardt, M.D., Ph.D., medical director of the Santa Fe Pain Center in Santa Fe, New Mexico. Dr. Klinghardt, who is a Board Certified Diplomate in the pain management specialties of neurological and orthopaedic medicine, uses reconstructive therapy on a regular basis. His report came to us October 5, 1989, just as we were completing the first draft of this chapter.

Dr. Klinghardt wrote:

"Walter Glengood is a 55-year-old real estate broker who runs a very successful business in Santa Fe. Over twenty years ago he developed neck pain, with no apparent trauma occurring at the time. Initially he saw several orthopedic surgeons, several neurosurgeons, and an osteopath. He was treated with many courses of physical therapy, osteopathic manipulation, and anti- inflammatory medication. At the time of his difficulty, a myelogram was suggested to him [by one of the neurosurgeons] in order to rule out a spinal tumor being present or a significant disc herniation as the source of trouble. He refused to have that myelogram done. In the later course of his treatments he sought out the services of chiropractors, acupuncturists, and several other health care providers. All of the different modalities appeared to give him slight relief lasting for a few hours or, at best, a few days at a time. There was no significant pain-relieving breakthrough for him. Over the years his neck pain became increasingly more severe.

"Eventually he underwent a CAT scan [computerized axial tomograph] and an MRI scan [magnetic resonance imaging], and since then he had not gone to see a regular medical doctor. But then Walter Glengood consulted me in the fall of 1988. He presented me with a list of signs and symptoms that included severe restriction of motion of the cervical spine with extreme tenderness over the cervical facet joints and over the lower interspinous spaces. He was suffering from chronic severe headaches which were with him almost every day. He admitted to treating himself with aspirin and extra strength Tylenol™.

"I could find no hard neurological findings indicating pressure on the spinal cord (cervical myelopathy) or pressure on

150

one of the cervical nerve roots.

"I explained to the patient that it would be good to obtain an MRI and a fresh set of x-rays before initiating treatment. He said that he had had so many x-rays in the past that he would be willing to accept more, or an MRI, only if I felt that it would make a large difference in my treatment. I explained to him that since his pain had been present in the neck for over twenty years, it was unlikely to be a malignant spinal tumor. It was most likely that MRI would show one or several degenerated cervical discs.

"We settled our differences in diagnostic procedure with a compromise. The decision was for me to treat him several times with reconstructive therapy. If there was no progress in his condition, we would then do an MRI.

"The following treatment was performed: I gave him manipulation of the cervical spine (mobilization of the cervical spine under strong traction) on the first day, followed thereafter by five treatment series of injections with proliferants. The five sets of injections were given one week apart with 20 cc of the Ongley solution [as described in the California placebo-controlled double-blind study] on each occasion.

"After the fifth treatment, Walter Glengood was completely free of pain. His range of motion had dramatically increased. Rotation to either side [turning his head] was approximately 45 degrees before the treatment and 90 degrees after the treatment.

"This patient has been completely painfree for eight months. I do not expect any relapses in his condition. He has a bright future. If there were to be a significant relapse, I would probably give him one more treatment with reconstructive therapy."

Chapter Ten

Shoulder Disability and TMJ Syndrome

Ever since he was struck by mortar fire and thrown 200 feet down a Korean hill, Frank Wilson, now 51 and a former Milwaukee bus driver, has suffered with serious degenerative joint disease in the cervical spine, right shoulder, and low back. He was first hospitalized overseas for a month and then spent more weeks in a hospital bed stateside. Still feeling intense pain in his neck, he was medically discharged from the service and receives disability pay.

In the years that followed, Frank sought help from many medical experts at Veterans Administration hospitals, including orthopedic surgeons, neurologists, and physiatrists (specialists in physical medicine) Then he attempted to find help from alternative medical practioners such as osteopaths, chiropractors, a cranial therapist, physical therapists, occupational therapists, and more. He stopped keeping count of the number after his list exceeded twenty-eight health professionals of one kind or another. No type of therapy seemed to relieve his deep-seated shoulder pain, constant neck pain, repeated migraine headaches, prolonged general achiness along his spine, lack of endurance, and quick fatigue. Orthopedic surgeons at the VA recommended a spinal fusion, but Frank refused. He knew that spinal surgery was frequently unsuccessful.

"I couldn't play with my kids," Frank told us. "I just had to cut back with any activity that I tried. My whole family suffered because of my body aches and pains. My shoulder was so painful that I couldn't tie my own shoelaces. Riding in a car, I felt every little bump in the road. After walking or standing, I would have to sit down and rest. It was a terrible blow to my masculine ego to see my wife and children performing my household chores like mowing the lawn or shoveling snow off the sidewalk simply because it caused me too much pain to do these jobs. Sometimes I managed OK by taking strong pain pills prescribed by the medical doctor or by receiving manipulations from osteopathic physicians or chiropractors. These treatments helped but never really changed the course of searing pain from my torn shoulder or the headaches and achiness in my back."

The ex-soldier's pain and disability lasted thirty-three years before he was referred to the Milwaukee Pain Clinic and Metabolic Research Center by Michael P. Szatalowicz, D.C. of the Atlas Chiropractic Center, located near the pain clinic. Dr. Szatalowicz is a superb orthogonal chiropractor who uses a gentle form of manipulation technique. However, when he recognized the seriousness of this patient's neck problem, the chiropractor came to believe that Frank Wilson would receive more effective relief from Dr. Faber's ministrations.

At first Frank considered Dr. Szatalowicz's referral just another dead end, but he went through with the visits to Dr. Faber anyway. In astonishment, then gratification, and eventually joy, he found that this reconstruction treatment was exactly what he and his wife had been praying to find.

At the Milwaukee Pain Clinic x-ray examination and clinical findings revealed that the patient had severe arthritic disease through the neck and low back with marked multiple cervical disc degeneration. Worse than that, he had tearing of nearly all of the shoulder ligaments and tendons, especially the coracohumeral and the coracoacromial ligaments and the subscapularis, supraspinatus, and infraspinatus muscles. Because of these rotator cuff tears, his humerus, clavical, and

153

scapula were perpetually in a state of near-dislocation. No wonder that his right shoulder brought him awful pain everytime he turned the bus steering wheel.

Additionally, his metabolic status was in bad shape. He first needed biological medical care to correct his nutritional failings. Dr. Faber admonished Frank that he must get rid of the toxic elements in his colon and pull himself away from smoking, drinking, eating fatty hamburgers and gobbling hot dogs as a quick lunch. For him, it was no more pizza, ice cream, soda pop, white flour baked goods, fast foods at restaurants, convenience foods at home, and other processed garbage that he usually put into his body. Frank couldn't see the wisdom of discontinuing the junk food diet that he always had eaten — his favorite stuff like beer and pretzels in front of the television set, potato chips as he drove the bus, or fish and chips with a quart of coffee. Still, he went along with the doctor's "improved lifestyle" recommendations. He had done everything else to get rid of his neck and shoulder trouble, hadn't he? His diet improved markedly. He ate unsweetened yogurt, fresh vegetables, fresh fruits, whole grains and more raw foods like salad. His wife bought their food in the health food store, and her entire family benefited from the enhanced nutrition. He drank coffee substitutes made of figs and cereal grains, and he was put on herbal bowel cleansers. He also took many nutritional supplements to build up his immune system.

It was a few weeks before Dr. Faber started reconstructive therapy at the base of his skull and to the tendons and ligaments in his neck. Since the shoulder is closely tied to the cervical spine's anatomy, it is necessary to make this part of the body strong before starting elsewhere. The patient responded well to the first injection treatment. Right away the veteran reported to his spouse marked improvement in the way he could bend his neck. The intensity of his headaches decreased steadily with each neck joint reconstruction. After twelve treatments, Frank's headaches were completely gone. Driving the bus, he found that he could turn his neck in any direction without restriction. Before reconstructive therapy, he had been forced to turn his entire body to see to the left side. However, his right shoulder still gave him pain.

After the cervical region was corrected and his neck impairments had disappeared, reconstructive ligament and tendon injections were given to the whole area of the shoulder on a weekly basis. As he approached the sixth month of weekly injections, his shoulder was improved to the point that he did not feel any pain at all. The torn ligaments had been reinforced with new connective tissue stimulated to form by the proliferant irritants.

Frank reported that he was able to accomplish much more each day without feeling fatigue. The quality of his life grew so fulfilling that he thought he could even quit driving a bus and start toward his dream of establishing a woodworking hobby shop. That's what he eventually did. He took his savings, and an early retirement pension and opened a small shop. Today you can visit him as he handcrafts fancy furniture and sells woodcrafter supplies in Waukesha, Wisconsin.

The Shoulder-Arm Complex

The shoulder is constructed so that the humerus (upper arm bone) swings from a movable base formed by the scapula behind and the clavicle in front together with the muscles and ligaments which form the capsule. Within this capsule the ball-shaped head of the humerus fits into the cavity of the glenoid fossa of the scapula. The glenoid fossa is larger than the head of the humerus. A fibrocartilaginous ring further enlarges the articular surface so that the humerus head is allowed greater freedom of movement. In payment for this great freedom of movement you depend on viable ligaments and strong musculature to keep the shoulder joint intact if you place strenuous demands on it.

As indicated in Figure 20, depicting the normal shoulder, the capsular ligament ties the head of the humerus into the glenoid fossa, and the joint is reinforced above by the coracohumeral and the coracoacromial ligaments. These ligaments are inadequate to keep the shoulder joint in its normal position. Consequently, the support of the shoulder joint also depends on the tone of the surrounding muscles. The front and side portions of the capsule are the weakest. When throwing a block in football or attempting to catch a heavy object, you hold your arms out with the humerus rotated outward. This places the greatest stress on the capsule. The strongest position of the shoulder is with the humerus held downward and inwardly rotated. Figure 20 also shows that the capsular ligament is firm at the distal portion and loose at the proximal part to permit freedom of movement.

When Frank Wilson was blasted out of his fox hole, his shoulder was not damaged by the explosion. Rather, the ligaments were splintered and torn apart, as shown in Figure 21, by his being thrown down the hillside. For thirty-three years afterward he suffered with chronic joint pain because nothing was ever done to make his ligaments heal or to form new connective tissue. Of the more than twenty-eight health professionals from whom he purchased services, none of them were trained, or perhaps even aware of reconstructive therapy.

The end product of injecting proliferants for production of new connective tissue (cicatrix) is seen in Figure 22. The patient's fibroblasts have been stimulated causing tissue growth. The result is that the right shoulder is actually stronger, firmer, and more effective in its movements than before Frank's war injury. Pain is no longer a factor in his life, because the inflammation that he lived with every day is completely eliminated. Not being ragged, relaxed, and malfunc-

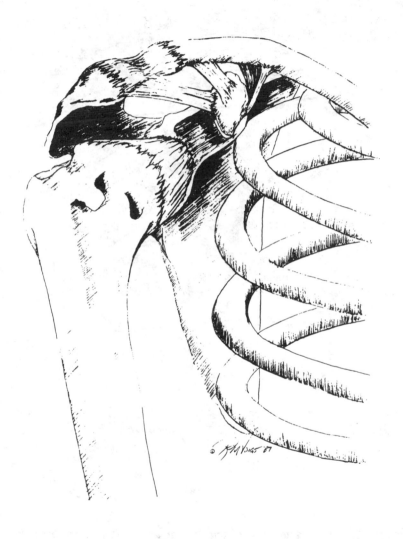

Figure 20. The stabilizing ligaments of a normal shoulder.

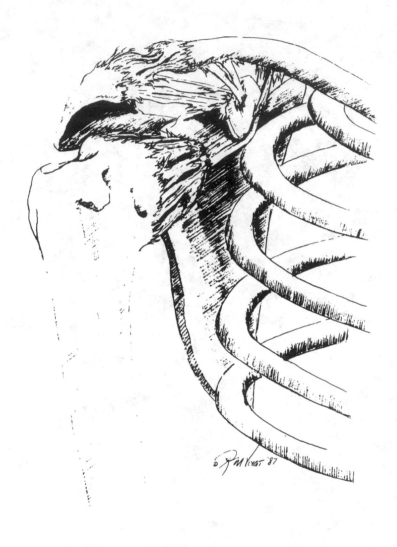

Figure 21. Torn and loosened ligaments that are producing instability in a shoulder.

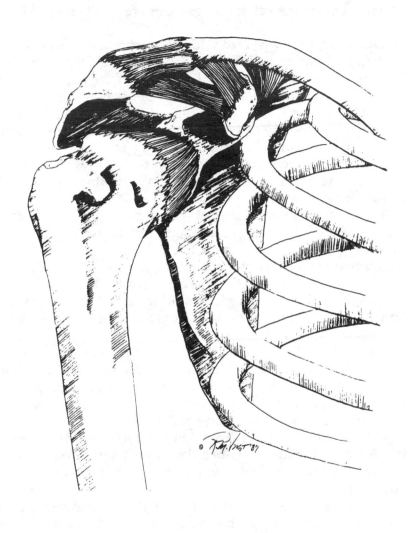

Figure 22. Reconstructed ligaments that are stronger and firmer, allowing the shoulder to function normally.

tional anymore, the veteran's ligaments are finally restored.

Rotator Cuff Tear Resolved with Reconstructive Therapy

Ralph Hampton is a fireman from Kansas City, Missouri. He has worked at this occupation for over 35 years without incident. About two years ago while he was using a heavy piece of equipment in a rescue, the equipment jammed causing a violent jerk to Ralph's left arm. It felt to him like he tore some tissue inside the shoulder. He consulted the fire department's orthopedic surgeon who took x-rays and a CAT scan and prescribed rest, physical therapy, ice treatments, and medication.

The orthopedist's treatment program didn't work, and Ralph suffered daily pain. He could not use the arm without increasing discomfort in his shoulder. The fire department doctor had another set of X-ray films taken, this time with dye applied into the shoulder. This uncovered a rotator cuff tear. The rotator cuff is the muscle that brings about rotation of the arm in the shoulder socket. Tearing takes place in the tendons and ligaments that are situated deep within the shoulder joint.

The orthopedic surgeon said, of course, that the "only" way to fix it was with an operation. Ralph's daughter, who is an experienced nurse, told him, "Dad, don't go through the surgery. I've seen so many people who have not gotten any better from having it, and many got worse."

Ralph went for a second opinion at a medical school hospital. After evaluation, the specialist confirmed, "You have a rotator cuff trear; the 'only' way you'll get better is to have an operation."

Remembering his daughter's advice, the fireman decided to travel across the country to one of the world's most famous clinics. After a physical examination, more x-rays, and reviews of his previous x-ray films and scans, he again heard he had a rotator cuff tear and that surgery was necessary. By this time

Ralph had suffered with shoulder pain for over a year and had been unable to return to work. He went ahead and scheduled the operation.

Just prior to his surgery, a relative of Ralph's said that the Milwaukee Pain Clinic used a special technique for shoulder problems like the one affecting him. She suggested that he look into it. He scheduled an appointment with Dr. Faber who examined the man's shoulder, checked all of his x-ray films. Dr. Faber determined that if Ralph's body had good healing ability, he would benefit from reconstructive therapy. He underwent a series of injections with proliferating solutions.

After his first treatment, Ralph noted a marked improvement in the way he was able to move his shoulder and arm. Contrary to the doctor's instructions, he believed himself to be doing so much better, he used a pick-ax to break up and repair his driveway. This heavy labor produced a setback.

Dr. Faber explained that many times after a patient starts to feel better, he or she does want to do too much too soon. Since reconstructive therapy is a building treatment within the tissues and takes time for the tissue growth to reach full strength, heavy work should be avoided until the area is recovered. With reconstructive therapy for the rotator cuff tear, the main effect is strengthening the tendons and ligaments in the area. Only the side effect is less pain. Usually a patient notices loss or lessening of pain early in the treatment process. Nonetheless, it takes time to build new tissue. Ralph resumed treatment and fully recovered with only a few more sets of proliferant injections. He went back to work.

Dr. Ellis Browning Helps a Fellow Physician

In the latter part of 1975, long-practiced reconstruction therapist Ellis V. Browning, M.D. of Yuma, Arizona helped one of his medical colleagues who had been suffering with unrelieved shoulder pain for nearly three years. This 60-year-old, physician had gone through every therapy in the book: physiotherapy, cortisone injections, cortisone by mouth, non-steroidal anti- inflammatory agents, anesthetic injections, prolonged rest, and more. Absolutely nothing helped. There wasn't even a clearcut diagnosis as to the cause of his condition.

Dr. Browning determined that the true disorder troubling this fellow physician consisted of overly loose shoulder ligaments: the coraco-acromial ligament, the transverse humeral ligament, and probably others.

"I gave him three reconstruction treatments with proliferating solutions directly into those ligamentous structures," Dr. Browning said. "They were spaced one week apart for each injection series. The doctor has remained painfree until now, ten years later."

The same physician returned to Dr. Browning in 1984 for more reconstructive therapy. "He jumped from a bulldozer and sustained contusion and pain in his right hip which stayed with him for six months until he decided to seek my services. A single set of reconstructiive therapeutic injections into the posterior hip capsule helped him immediately. He has remained free of hip discomfort for five years, until the present," said Dr. Browning.

The Out of Joint Jaw

Living in Ames, Iowa for all of her life, Amelia Hartford, age 68, suffered for about 13 years from Temporomandibular joint dysfunction — commonly referred to as TMJ sydrome. At first it had not hurt but only produced an annoying popping sound now and then. It intensified after a few years, and then pain and aching in the jaw started. She felt like her jaw bone was out of joint.

Mrs. Hartford sought professional help first from her family dentist who gave her a splint to wear over her teeth. That helped, but the popping sound worsened and got louder, especially when she chewed. At other times her jaw got sore if she spoke too much. Eventually she quit eating Iowa corn on the cob and meat, such as steak, that required chewing. Moreover, she became a kind of "silent" conversationalist and just kept her mouth shut.

The next time Mrs. Hartford asked for help was from an oral surgeon in Des Moines. He said that her Temporomandibular joint had become so unstable that surgery was the only way to give her relief. He added, "However, there is no guarantee that it would get better or stay better after you've had the operation." This confused her. She didn't know what to do to get the problem corrected.

A telephone conversation with her sister, Mrs. Annie Filbert, revealed that Mrs. Filbert's neighbor had found relief from the same type of TMJ problem. So, Amelia Hartford visited her sister who lives southwest of Fullerton, Nebraska. The sisters made an appointment for Mrs. Hartford with Arthur Dowell, M. D. Dr. Dowell informed Mrs. Hartford that her neck as well as the jaw should be treated. He explained how the neck supports the jaw, the head, and all the special sense organs of the eyes, ears, nose, and mouth. Mrs. Amelia Hartford was anxious to do anything to rid herself of this chronic out-of-joint jaw. She visited Mrs. Filbert's house weekly so she could keep her appointment with Dr. Dowell. Each time she underwent reconstructive therapy she noticed a little more improvement in the way her jaw felt. It didn't get out of joint, popping noices stopped, and pain disappeared. It took a few months — about 14 visits to Dr. Dowell — but the boring pains and deep aches finally left her entirely.

Mrs. Hartford said, "I really knew that I was free from my jaw nightmare when I ate like a hog one day after the last visit for reconstructive therapy and the menu for me was thick steak and four pieces of sweet corn on the cob."

Temporomandibular Joint Dysfunction

For some TMJ, temporomandibular joint dysfunction, is as minor as a persistent but annoying click of the jaw. For others it is a debilitating, withering pain or a locking of the jawbone — a pain in the head, neck, even the back and shoulders. H. David Hall, D.D.S., chairman of the department of oral surgery at Vanderbilt University Medical Center in Nashville, Tennessee, explains that "TMJ occurs when the alignment of the hinged temporomandibular joint, which connects the lower jawbone with the bones forming the side and base of the skull, goes awry."

The imbalance is present in nearly two-thirds of the general population and is considered a common cause of pain in the jaw joint; however, only a small proportion of those people actually feel symptoms serious enough to seek treatment, Dr. Hall said.

The jaw joint is similar to the knee, and has a disc that with stress can become dislocated. TMJ can occur at any age — as early as 10 years old or as late as 70 years — and is most often seen in those who grind their teeth. Stress, bad posture, head trauma, and even crooked teeth also have been blamed for causing the dysfunction.

Ever since Hippocrates, doctors have been finding and fixing ills of the hinge that joins jaw to cranium. But only for the past decade has TMJ syndrome come to be seen as a true health menace. One in five Americans, at least 50,000,000 people, says the American Dental Association, are hobbled by pain or other dysfunction of the TMJ. So insidious is this disorder that it robs athletes of power and afflicts ordinary mortals with everything from toothaches, headaches and backaches to hemorrhoids, scoliosis, and even schizophrenia. The symptomology is vast, varied, and vexatious.

164

To deal with this menace, TMJ clinics have sprung up around the country. Some dentists are even breaking jaws in hopes that changing bites will ease the pain. Kinesiologists are trying shoelifts to restore body equilibrium that TMJ troubles may destroy. Dietiticians are serving joint-saving soft-food diets. Calling TMJ a switchboard for nerve impulses throughout the body, chiropractors are manipulating to assuage disruptive joints. Iridologists are wide-eyed over the possibilities TMJ dysfunction opens for their whole-body theory of therapy. Oral surgeons like Dr. Hall are applying jaw splints and performing surgery .

One oral surgical technique involves repositioning the disc and repairing the torn ligaments which originally held it in place. In patients with more serious symptoms such as a locked jaw, a condylotomy is done. This procedure involves cutting the bone just below the joint, which allows the top part of the lower jaw to move forward in a reduced position in relation to the disc, limiting its movement to prevent further stress. When the disc has been irreparably damaged, a meniscectomy, a surgical procedure that involves the removal of the disc and ligaments in the area, is chosen.

All this is a case of a long-neglected health problem finally getting the respect and attention it is due. Needless to say, many of the treatments just mentioned, can be discarded in favor of just one highly effective procedure that works — reconstructive therapy. Unfortunately, few doctors and proportionately fewer patients having TMJ know about joint reconstruction for the jaw.

The Major Causes of TMJ Syndrome

Because he uses reconstructive therapy as a medical tool and reported to us on numerous and dramatic cases, we are furnishing you with another patient history of Ellis V. Browning, M.D. of Yuma, Arizona. Dr. Browning is Board Certified in Family Practice and a member of the American Osteopathic Academy of Sclerotherapy. He took care of Gladys Hobson, a 47-year-old diabetic housewife. The woman was experiencing left temporomandibular joint syndrome with pain radiating throughout the left side of her face and head. It remained unrelieved by non-steroidal anti-inflammatory drugs (NSAID) or by Decadron™ (corticosteroid) injections, the two standard modes of treatment to relieve pain from the condition. Being an uncontrolled diabetic, it would have been dangerous for Mrs. Hobson to undergo oral surgery.

One reconstructive therapeutic injection administered to Mrs. Hobson by Dr. Browning resolved her condition. Her TMJ syndrome went away permanently.

Why does the joint act up? Those who tangle with it suggest three general problems: emotional stress, mechanical pressure and bad bite.

What most people with TMJ syndrome have is too-tight jaw muscles, says oral surgeon Daniel L. Laskin, director of the TMJ and Facial Pain Center at the Medical College of Virginia. They get that way from stress-related muscle tension. Tight muscles around the joint — myofascial pain dysfunction, or MPD he calls it — causes most cases of TMJ disorder. The problem stems from years of jutting the jaw or clenching or grinding teeth, says Dr. Laskin — in short, habits of using the mouth to absorb stress.

Other TMJ experts say the primary trouble is malocclusion of the teeth, with or without muscle tension. The teeth and/or jaw are so poorly aligned that they impede natural movement of the temporomandibular joint. It gets battered every time the mouth opens and shuts. The malocclusion exponents correctly point out that over the years teeth may shift position or grind down slightly.Orthodontist Lawrence S. Harte, D.D.S., director of the New Jersey Center for Cranial Facial Pain in Livingston, New Jersey, explained that those who regularly spend hours on the phone, especially if they lean on a shoulder cradle, risk putting excess pressure on the TMJ. Moving the jawbone open and shut for talking or eating creates special hazards for the joint. It must bear the enormous forces of chewing and absorb the shock waves from nervous gritting of the teeth. Tension and spasm can grab the muscles that move the joint, and its inner cartilage disk can wear and tear. Also, unlike any other joint, the action of the TMJ is governed by outside forces: the condition and position of the teeth. The temporomandibular joint is unique, the only articulation of its type in the body.

Anatomy of the Temporomandibular Joint

Louis W. Schultz, M.D., D.D.S., of the Department of Surgery, The Presbyterian Hospital in Chicago and the University of Illinois, College of Medicine in Chicago, wrote that the jaw exerts up to 500 pounds of pressure per square inch. This joint has certain peculiarities which allows it to be too mobile. These peculiarities are:

(1) The body of the mandible is heavy and this stands the crushing strength, but the neck and head of the bone's condyle are light. This shows that these great forces must be muscularly balanced, and the TMJ does not take the major stress and strain. It is merely a guiding member to perfect articulation.

(2) The temporomandibular is one of twin joints located at either end of a horseshoe-shaped bone, the mandible.

(3) Its peculiar construction permits more free motion in all directions than is found in other joints.

(4) Both joints move through a similar pathway when in motion.

(5) Either one or both condyles may be removed and good function retained.

(6) One or both condyles may be fractured and healing per-

mitted with the condyle in almost any position, yet the resulting function will be practically normal.

(7) The condyles are rather loosely suspended in their sockets.

Hypermobility of the TMJ has it loose so that it can go into dysfunctional mini-dislocations. Typical causes of such dislocations are yawning, long dental sittings, extraction of teeth, manipulation of the patient's jaw while under general anesthesia, singing, sleeping with the head resting on the arm, injudicious use of mouth gags, congenital weakness of the joint's ligaments, a variety of accidents, and bad habits in the movements of the mandible.[1]

Dr. Schultz said that hypermobility is an all-inclusive term, meaning more motion than normal. He reported that he was able to correct chronic luxations and subluxations of the TMJ with intra- articular injections of a proliferating agent, sodium psylliate.[2] Through animal experments he also proved that the involved ligaments became thickened, and consequently stronger. Through clinical measurements, he was able to demonstrate an actual shortening of these structures.

Symptoms of TMJ Syndrome

In TMJ syndrome, pain may be constant or intermittent, localized in the region of the ear on either or both sides. As a rule, nevertheless, the pain settles into only one side of the jaw and occurs when the joint is used. It may be referred to other parts of the head on the same side, for example, the temple, cheek, mastoid, occiput, or neck.

Clicking or grating is frequently present during one or all three phases: opening, closing and exertion of pressure, as when the patient is chewing. In complete TMJ dislocation, the mouth is opened and cannot be closed by the individual. Locking of the jaws may occur when they are opened in loose articulation. The meniscus or fibrocartilaginous disc is usually responsible for this condition. In such instances it is caught and folded between the head of the condyle and the other articulating bone.

Mental and emotional anxiety is invariably affecting the patient suffering with TMJ syndrome. The dread of having the jaw dislocated, with locking or extreme pain, or both, induces a phobia.

John Sessions, D.O. Eliminates TMJ

Evelyn Pharos of Woodville, Texas, a friendly homemaker, age 72, became just such a phobic person when temporomandibular joint syndrome came upon her. Full of energy and always cooking for and giving to those about her, she began to notice a pain above her right upper dentures. She consulted her dentist, but he recognized nothing unusual. He told her to take an aspirin for her discomfort. However, the pain continued, worsened, and kept Mrs. Pharos in a state of emotional upset. By turns, she became depressed, anxious, neurotic, and started to speak of doing away with herself. Her jaw pain gave her no peace.

Eventually she brought her problem to John L. Sessions, D.O., who had built a reputation in and around the tiny town of Kirbyville, Texas where he is medical director of the Jasper County Medical Center. Dr. Sessions is skilled in the application of reconstructive therapy.

This osteopathic physician examined Mrs. Pharos and noted the area below the right maxillary sinus to be tender and somewhat swollen. He ordered a CAT scan of the patient. She was referred to an eye, ear, nose, and throat specialist who diagnosed a cyst growing in the bone on the right side of her jaw where the upper teeth should normally be. A biopsy proved the tumor noncancerous.

Mrs. Pharos was faced with disfiguring, painful surgery on

her upper jaw bone (the maxilla). It would be necessary to remove all or part of it. Dr. Sessions decided to try another tact first, something that has no side effects and was not contraindicated.

He used reconstructive therapy into the benign tumor in the patient's jaw bone. Mrs. Pharos considered it "a miracle" when after only three nearly painless injections of sodium morrhuate, her pain and swelling were completely alleviated. The problem just disappeared from her life.

Now two years later, Evelyn Pharos can wear her dentures, smile, and care for those about her without any recurrence of the tumor or pain in her upper jaw.

Dr. Faber reports success using reconstructive therapy for TMJ laxity. He adds that often TMJ involves multiple factors that all need to be addressed in order to resolve this situation. The dentist tends to concentrate on the factors within the nouth caused by a change in the height of the teeth. If dental work cannot correct the problem, osteopathic or chiropractic manipulation of the jaw may help.

TMJ can also be influenced by posture, stability of the spine, position of the spine, pelvis, or sacrum, or pronation of the foot. Weakness in the stylomandibular ligament can cause TMJ pain.

Small reconstruction injections into it's attachments on the mandible can produce marked improvements in TMJ pain and return proper function.

Another important factor in TMJ pain and dysfunction is scars and nerve problems. The profound effects that scars and nerve problems can have on the TMJ as well as on other areas of the body are explained in the book, also by Drs. Faber and Walker, *Instant Pain Relief*. This book can be obtained from the Milwaukee Pain Clinic for $15,00. Scars and nerve dysfunction cause a pulling on the tissue which can contribute to TMJ pain. The book has a chapter on head pain as well as two chapters on self-diagnosis and self-treatment. It also contains nearly 100 actual case histories.

Frequently hidden infections of the jaws and teeth can cause pain in the area of the TMJ. Often specially trained dentists and physicians are able to detect and treat them. For more information send a self-addressed stamped legal-size envelop to:

American Academy of Biological Dentistry
P. O. Box 856
Carmel Valley, California 93924

Metals in the teeth and mouth can generate tiny electrical currents and sometimes toxicities which can contribute to TMJ pain and dysfunction. For further information contact:

Huggins Diagnostic Center
P. O. Box 2589
Colorado Springs, CO 80901
1-800-331-2303

Chapter Eleven
Success with Proliferants
for Knee Trouble

An exponent and experienced therapist with injectible proliferants, Richard F. Leedy, D.O. of Woodbury, New Jersey, has been using them to correct his patients' joint problems for over thirty years. "Reconstructive therapy for knee trouble is highly successful," said Dr. Leedy. "It is a fine replacement for surgery on the very sensitive knee joint. With knee surgery's questionable after-effects in later years, any informed professional is given to wondering how much of the current operative procedures done on athletes could be avoided by first using adequate osteopathic evaluation and ligament repair readily available with reconstructive therapy.

"My colleagues in the Osteopathic Academy of Sclerotherapy and I have been using reconstructive therapy for many decades. The knee is one of those articulations which seems to respond especially well to injection with proliferants," Dr. Leedy said in an interview we conducted with him in the summer of 1987. "Torn knee ligaments readily grow new connective tissues so that eventually prior injury seems never to have happened.

"The best results can be achieved by the reconstruction therapist spreading the proliferant solution in small amounts throughout as much ligament tissue as possbile. Knees are sensitive, so the smallest possible size of needle is used. . . . The anesthesia takes effect quickly and little pain is felt. The solution is spread carefully throughout the capsular, coronary, and collateral ligaments," Dr. Leedy advised. He went on to describe the exact technique for a once-a-week injection schedule which "produces immediate pain relief plus fibro-osseous proliferative stimulation to create new ligament tissue support to the knee joint. . . . Many damaged knees that are apparently candidates for surgery can be rendered symptom-free and fully functional with this treatment," he said.

Dr. Leedy Treats Gouty Arthritis of the Knees

Dr. Leedy was visited by Alma Montgomery, 45, of Camden, New Jersey. She used a cane and experienced obvious distress from the pain in her knees, ankles, feet, and low back. Her troublesome knees were the site of her initial difficulties, she said, and the other joints of her body seemed to develop problems as her knees worsened.

Mrs. Montgomery reported that her chronic joint pains were becoming progressively worse. Once she had worked steadily as a waitress. "I made good tip money hustling at lunch and dinner, but I had to give up work almost a year ago because I couldn't maneuver among the tables anymore. My knees did me in. Now Manny and I (Manny is my husband) have got to manage on just his salary alone. He's an auto mechanic."

She was severely limited in movement most of the time and, as a result, had gained thirty pounds in the past year. She looked puffy and swollen.

Dr. Leedy supplied us with his clinical notes, in which he noted: "Clinical examination of Mrs. Montgomery reveals swelling and extremely painful soft tissue of the lower extremities, especially of the knees and low back. Laboratory examination of her blood chemistry was normal except for a high serum uric acid. X-ray examination does not reveal excessive joint degeneration in the lumbosacral and knee articulations.

"My diagnosis is gouty arthritis, ligament insufficiency of

173

both knees plus low back and general debilitation. Prognosis [the eventual outcome of treatment] is good if the following treatment program is followed: (1) prescribing of a high vitamin, low purine diet regimen, (2) giving her antigout medication, and (3) administering injections of proliferating agents plus local anesthetic into her lumbosacral ligaments [two separate areas] and into both knees. At each visit all four regions of pathology must receive mild proliferant injections."

Mrs. Montgomery was put on the dietary corrections, took oral medication against gout, and at the next visit — seven days later — began to receive weekly injections of reconstructive therapy solutions. The proliferants brought her immediate relief — at least by the next day when her initial joint stiffness wore off. She was overjoyed. A couple of visits later she threw away her cane.

"Results were gratifying," Dr. Leedy told us. "The patient lost weight steadily so as to relieve strain on the knee joints. They became free of pain most of the time. After ten weeks she was pain-free all of the time and able to resume her normal life pattern. She went back to work as a waitress where she had formerly been employed. Manny and Alma's weekly income doubled.

"As determined by my telephone call to her in preparation for this interview," said the osteopathic physician, "it's seven years later [remembering that our interview took place in mid-1987] and the recheck on her progress brought continuation of Mrs. Montgomery's happiness with reconstructive therapy. The patient said that no recurrence of chronic joint pain in her knees or other areas had ever taken place."

Anatomy of the Knee Joint

The knee joint is a bizarre blend of paradoxes. It is free, yet firm, stable, yet versatile, massive, yet shapely. Most of the complex of rotations in all three planes which result from the interactions of movements of the upper extremity upon the spine in walking and running are transferred through the hip and femur to the knees. The rotary motion of the pelvis also turns the femur against the tibia at the knee. The oblique set of the femur above the knee causes the weight of the body to be transferred to the knee in an angular position. These stresses and strains are absorbed very well by a competent knee joint. The forces directed toward the ankle and foot through the tibia and fibula in walking and running, because of adjustments in the knee joint, are, for the most part, in the sagittal (straight line from front to back) plane.

The absorption of stresses and strains is only a secondary function of the knee. Its primary function make the lower leg move.

The knee joint meets the rotatory stresses imparted by the femur by means of strong ligaments binding the bones together. The knee joint is surrounded by fascia, tendons, and ligaments. Its front portion is bound by the capsular and patellar ligaments which allow an extreme range of flexion. The back portion is joined by the short popliteal ligament which checks hyperextension of the joint. Sideward displacement is prevented to the inside by the tibial and to the outside by the fibular collateral ligaments. In the middle of the knee joint lie the anterior and posterior cruciate ligaments, crossing each other like the lines of the letter X . The anterior cruciate ligament checks rotation inward. Outward rotation tends to uncross and relax the cruciates. They bind the femur and tibia together and prevent extreme motion of the tibia forward and backward and inward in rotation (see Figure 23).

Also seen in Figure 23 are the semilunar menisci, two crescent- shaped cartilages that are thickest at the edges and attached to the inside of the joint, and are free at the outside borders. The relatively small surfaces of the head of the tibia are deepened for the articulation with large condyles of the

175

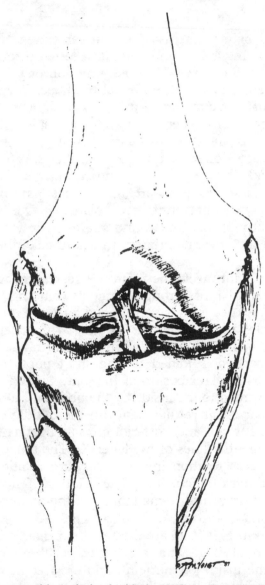

Figure 23. The normal knee depicted with the patellar removed so as to show taut ligaments on either side of the bones and internal crossed ligaments.

femur by the two semilunar fibrocartilages — the menisci.

.The upper and lower surfaces of each meniscus are concave and are invested with a smooth synovial membrane which serves to lubricate the knee joint. Motion in the knee thus takes place as an articulation between the condyles of the femur and the upper surfaces of the semilunar menisci and the condyles of the tibia and the lower surfaces of the menisci. During the beginning of a deep knee bend from an erect standing position, the articulating surfaces of the condyles of the femur rock backward over the menisci above the corresponding surfaces of the condyles of the tibia. After 20 degrees of flexion the type of motion of the articulating surfaces of the femur and tibia changes from a rocking motion to a gliding motion over the surfaces of the menisci. The knee is designed for two separate functions. When the leg is flexed less than 20 degrees, the joint is stable due to the restrictions of the surrounding ligaments. When the knee is flexed beyond 20 degrees, the reinforcing ligaments in the rear of the leg are relaxed because the condyles are closed together in the rear. The flexed joint becomes loose and free for axial rotations. The flexed knee is not adapted to weight-bearing functions.

The semilunar menisci are commonly torn or loosened due to a severe blow or twist. If one meniscus is removed as in surgery, the other becomes the major weight-bearing surface and its susceptibility to injury is increased. In giving way to the tramatic blow or twist, the menisci absorb some of the force. With the minisci removed this safety factor is absent and a severe blow or twist is more likely to rupture the ligaments or shatter the articulating surfaces of the bones.

The total range of motion in the knee joint is 130 degrees from slight overextension to full flexion. With the knee in right angle flexion the range of motion from outward rotation to inward rotation is 50 to 60 degrees.

The inner lining of the knee joint is called synovium. Rheumatoid arthritis and other diseases can cause the synovium to overgrow abnormally. The overactive synovium produces pain, swelling, and can actually destroy the articular cartilage.

Crippling Knee Arthritis Resolved
with Reconstructive Therapy

At age 86, Jonathan Angstrom of Antigo, Wisconsin was overweight and suffered with severe degenerative joint disease of both knees. His wife Julia began to believe that he would have to spend his last years in a nursing home separated from her. She was finding it increasingly difficult to lift him from the wheel chair and put him on the toilet. The wife had trouble dressing her husband, too, and sometimes he would spend the day only partially clothed.

Fifteen years ago the first serious pains and aching began. The pain was so disabling that Jonathan started using a cane. At times his knees would just give out. The cane gave him more confidence, so he continued to perform small personal functions for himself. But a few years later Julia's husband had to start using crutches. He never went outside anymore.

Another few years later, the pressures on his weakened knee joints forced Jonathan to employ a walker. That was in 1983. Then, in the spring of 1985, he was confined to a wheelchair. It was at that time that Julia found he was getting so heavy. The effort of moving him from the bed to the chair to the commode was breaking her down.

The worse that Jonathan got the more household duties she assumed. For the last decade she had essentially been doing all of the household duties. Thinking back, she states that the time since he started using the walker was the worst because he couldn't get up from a chair without rocking and straining. She would have to bend and help him stand up.

Sometimes his knees would give out and he fell down. She could no longer hold up her husband's weight, and it was at this point both of them knew something more had to be done.

Over a period of seven months, Julia took Jonathan to at least half-a-dozen specialists including rheumatologists, orthopedists, internists, and other medical experts in private practice, plus a university hospital and an advanced medical research facility at which new arthritis modalities were investigated. Nothing did the job for the man. It took time, much effort, and lots of money. They went through the balance of their retirement savings in paying for the diagnostic tests, prescription medicines, and various other items not covered by Medicare.

Julia Angstrom eventually learned that the Milwaukee Pain Clinic offered a technique that strengthens ligaments, tendons and joints. She was a bit skeptical at first as she had never heard of such a treatment before. Would it help Jonathan's osteoarthritis of the knees, she wondered? Nonetheless, conferring together, they decided to take the 200-mile drive in deep snow from Antigo to Milwaukee and give the services a try. It was the first week of January, 1986.

Before any treatment, Jonathan's laboratory test results and X-rays were evaluated at the Clinic. Dr. Faber found that the patient did, indeed, have severe deforming degenerative joint arthritis — osteoarthritis — of both knees due to physical, chemical, and emotional stresses and overweight. He also found a number of toxicities and nutritional imbalances in the elderly man. Part of his obvious chemical stress came from Jonathan's terrible diet.

The patient was placed on an improved diet, plus nutritional supplements and given intravenous nutritional and mineral replacement infusions to detoxify and balance his biochemical system. He was prescribed herbal laxatives and fiber to help clean out his poisoned colon. The Angstroms were disap-

179

pointed that the "magic" injection treatments that had brought them this distance from home were not given to Jonathan's knees during that first visit. They half-way hoped that he would go dancing out of Milwaukee in just one consultation with the doctor.

At the next visit when it was apparent to Dr. Faber that Julia had her husband cooperating in the program of detoxification and nutritional buildup he had prescribed, the physician made his first attempt at reconstructing Jonathan's osteoarthritic and deformed bowed knees.

Degenerative Arthritis of the Knees

Osteoarthritis or degenerative arthritis of the knees often begins in middle age and progresses as wear and tear takes place in the joints. Sometimes it occurs earlier, as a result of injuries or excessive stress and strain that takes place in youth, especially those traumas entailed in sports and occupations. Football knee, soccer ankle, pitcher's elbow, policeman's heel, march fracture, and dancer's foot are examples of precursors to osteoarthritis. Frequently these early injuries are the source of degenerative joint diseases later in life.

Typically, a ligamentous tear at the fibro-osseous junction of the medial collateral ligament (see Figure 24) is the beginning of degenerative arthritis of the knee. It may come from a simple twist as from taking a wrong step off a ladder or from disembarking from a slippery boat deck. Even such a minor injury could start the inflammatory process for osteoarthritis.

Pathology set up in osteoarthritis of the knees involves the pads of cartilage — the menisci — that cover the ends of the long leg bones gradually become worn away, allowing the femur's condyles and the tibia's head to rub together. This causes swelling and inflammation of the capsule surrounding the knee joint and produces pain or tenderness in the muscles and ligaments that move it. Such inflammation makes the

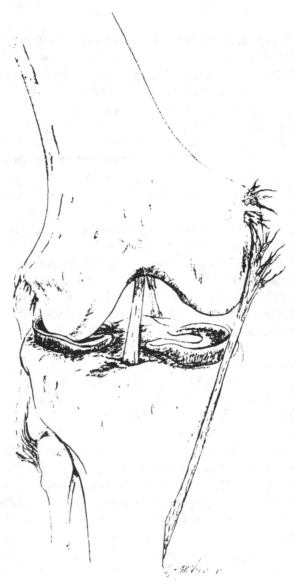

Figure 24. A knee damaged by a ligamentous tear at the fibro-osseous junction of its medial collateral ligament.

joint stiff, and in time joint movement may be restricted or lost entirely. More than that, and probably of greater importance, is that minor trauma that you might have sustained early on. The torn medial collateral ligament hurts, and the body comes to its own defense to try and limit motion in the injured area. The fibrocytes (bone-forming cells) bring calcium deposits to the traumatized knee to act as a mechanism of splinting. Over time, without appropriate correction of the torn ligaments, the calcium deposition becomes permanently established in the form of solid bubble-like lipping and spurring components along the edges of the knee articulation (as shown in Figure 25). Such hard calcium deposition to restrict joint motion is the actual arthritic result.

That is what happened to Jonathan Angstrom's two knees. He was filled with what is known in medicine as "metastatic calcium," meaning transportation of calcium ions from the blood stream to the joints where it does not belong. Yet this marvelous new-old treatment was just what the patient needed and the doctor ordered.

Solving Arthritis of the Knee with Reconstructive Therapy

Dr. Faber solved his patient's double arthritic knee problems with reconstructive therapy. The main effect of injecting proliferating solutions into the knee joint is to increase its strength and endurance. The injection solution does not take away existing arthritis. Metastatic calcium is too well-established for that to occur, and is as hard as any bone. Instead, the pain goes away because the metabolic inflammation is dissipated and is replaced with temporary local inflammation.

Reconstruction of the knee joint is similar to having bloodless surgery. The healing is stimulated by placing the proliferating agent — perhaps sodium morrhuate, a distilled pharmaceutical grade of cod liver fish oil — or some other biological stimulant precisely at the area of the tear or laxity

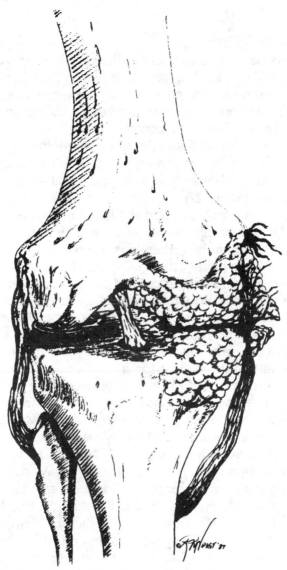

Figure 25. Tearing of the medial collateral ligament of the knee brings on chronic instability, resulting in loss of cartilage height, constant friction, and eventual arthritic spurring.

(see Figure 26).

This precisely-placed irritation dilates the blood vessels and signals fibroblastic healing cells to travel to the weakened area and lay down protein to permanently strengthen the impaired ligaments. The knee joint discontinues wobbling on its overly lax ligaments because they become strongly supportive of the joint. New connective tissue develops at the injection site and bridges the gap between the torn ligamentous portion and its insertion into the bone — in this case the lateral condyle of the femur (see Figure 27).

Jonathan Angstrom recalled the first time his left knee was injected. Dr. Faber injects one knee at a time and then both knees. For Jonathan, he remembers, it wasn't a marvelous experience, and the patient didn't fly out of the clinic under his own power either. He was pushed in the wheelchair by one of the Milwaukee Pain Clinic nurses. Their ride home to Antigo was uneventful because the anesthetic portion of the proliferating solution still was in effect.

He states that after the anesthetic wore off, his injected left knee felt stiff and swelled for a day or two. But then he noticed a lot more strength in the left knee and less pain. He compared it to the other knee that felt the same old weak, inflamed way it always had. He wished his Milwaukee appointment would be sooner than five days away. He wanted his right knee injected, as well.

Dr. Faber says that Jonathan's and Julia's determination was an important factor for success of the treatment. Jonathan travelled some 200 miles each week to obtain this treatment, and he followed the doctor's advice exactly. During the healing phase, he dropped forty pounds just by eating less refined carbohydrates, reducing his intake of fatty foods, and improving his bowel habits.

Steadily over the ensuing weeks, Jonathan noticed an improvement in strength in his knees. He moved from using a

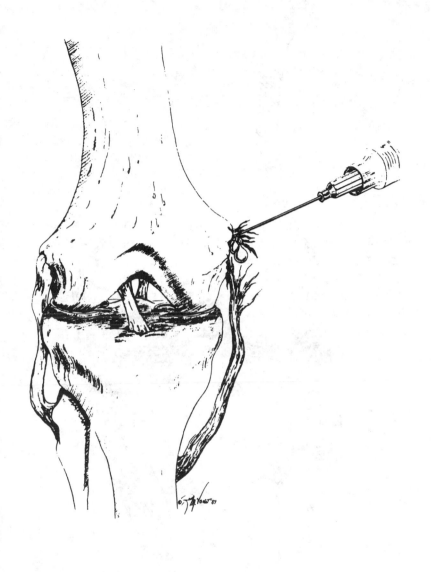

Figure 26. The precise injection area for torn medial collateral ligament of the knee.

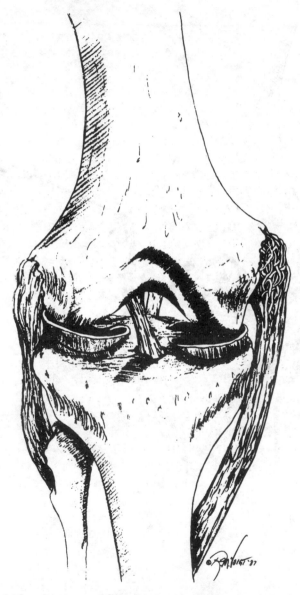

Figure 27. Reconstructed medial collateral ligament of the knee.

wheelchair and a walker to using only crutches. In April of 1987 he got up and walked without any assistance. Tears welled in Julia's eyes as the two of them realized he had succeeded in getting back his independence. They could continue to live out their lives without thoughts of a nursing home.

Jonathan continued his treatment and, in June 1987 he started mowing the lawn and using the roto-tiller in the garden. He went shopping for groceries with Julia, too. Jonathan has completed three seasons of mowing his own lawn, and he has celebrated his ninetieth birthday at the time of this writing. He wants to celebrate his 80th wedding anniversary with his bride when he is 100 years old. Stating that since he can walk again his life is worth more, he walks everywhere and gets up from a chair independently without aid. Do you wish to see what Jonathan Angstrom looks like? See Figure 27a, a gift photograph presented to Dr. Faber by the Angstroms.

A Clinical Study Proving Injured
Knees Benefit from the Treatment

Reconstructive therapy for arthritic and other painful joints, tendons and ligaments is the one sure means of alleviating joint inflammation. Studies proving its effects have been published.[1] Injuries to the knee are particularly responsive to joint reconstruction, and this was proven in a 1988 clinical study published in *Manual Medicine*. Conducted by five physicians and analyzed by a statistician, the study took place over a nine- month period for proliferant injection repair of the posterior and anterior cruciate and the medial and lateral collateral ligaments of impaired knees. Thirty patients presented themselves with knee pain but five knees in four patients were selected for study and correction because of substantial and reproducible ligament instability.[2] One of the hallmarks of a good clinical study is that it is reproducible by other doctors in other locations. For reprints of the study to

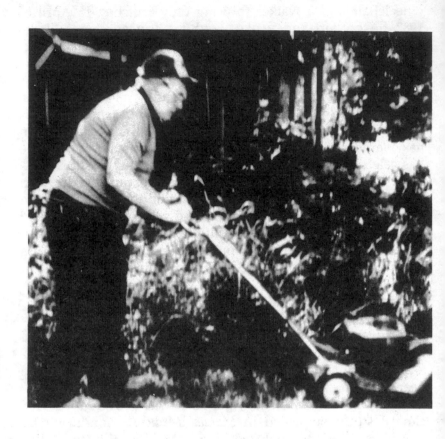

Figure 27a. After experiencing fifteen years of severe degenerative arthritis in the knees that required him to use crutches, a walker, and a wheelchair, 90-year-old Jonathan Angstrom of Antigo, Wisconsin is shown in a photograph mowing his lawn. Mr. Angstrom's knee problem was completely resolved by the physician's use of permanent, non-surgical reconstructive therapy, once again allowing this patient the independence that he had as a young man.

188

be described here, make your request accompanied by a self-addressed, stamped (45 cents in stamps) legal-size envelope to Thomas A. Dorman, M.D., 1041 Murray Avenue, San Luis Obispo, California 93401, USA.

The patients underwent multiple proliferating injections to achieve joint reconstruction. Subjective symptoms indicated by the patients were recorded at the beginning and end of the study, and objective symptoms of ligament stability were measured by a commercially available computerized instrument, the Genucom, produced by FARO Medical Technologies, Inc. of Montreal, Quebec Canada. The Genucom measuring device consists of a chair equipped with a six-component force platform and a six-degree of freedom electrogoniometer. With computer-integrated force and motion measurements, a standardized series of clinical laxity tests can be performed. Prior studies have compared clinical testing with objective tests[3] and such findings have been reproduced.[4]

Reconstructive therapy for knees works most effectively when interstitial rupture of collagen fibers within the substance of ligaments produces elongation and thus dysfunction. Also there should be repeated provocation of an inflammatory reaction within the ligament so as to induce fibroblastic hyperplasia [the increased production and growth of normal fibroblast cells] and the laying down of new collagen. As stated previously, collagen is a protein that makes up the prinicpal constituent of the white fibrous connective tissue that occurs in ligaments, cartilage, and tendons. It is relatively inelastic but has a high tensile strength. Consequently, healing of the involved ligaments will be achieved in the presence of normal active movement.

In the *Manual Medicine* study, the patients suffered from the conditions just described. No systemic or general complications occurred in the subjects under investigation. Sometimes an effusion of fluid and swelling did develop after a proliferant injection.

The laxity of unstable knees in this study group reduced quite a bit. All patients demonstrated improvement in measurable objective data. In addition, their subjective improvement and activity level became quite apparent. The four patients having five damaged knees were happy with the improved function. The study results, although performed on a small number of patients, were encouraging and provide the scientific format for further research. Such research was carried out by the same investigators the year before.[5] However, they look for other investigators practicing their same disciplines in rheumatology, orthopedics, and internal medicine to duplicate their results so as to confirm to the general medical community that reconstructive therapy is a superior treatment for chronic joint pain.

Knee Injuries Among Athletes

What do professional athletes Joan Benoit, Steve Mahre, and Mary Lou Retton have in common? Each has won major athletic competitions despite suffering serious difficulties with their knees. They have what might be called a "trick knee."

The trick knee is a disorder often encountered in young athletes. It means a knee that is easily strained because the cartilage or ligaments have been weakened by a previous injury. It goes out again from time to time. The injury will have occurred on either side of the knee and produce a tear in one or both of the cartilages lying between the two major bones. The ligaments are overly stretched or torn. Even so, the knee can function normally until a bit of the torn cartilage gets caught between the joint's surfaces, causing it to lock or making the knee suddenly give way. That's the "trickiness" of this injury. A trick knee may be helped by wearing a bandage, or it may be permanently corrected with reconstructive therapy.

Anterior cruciate ligament injuries occur predominantly during noncontact sports. Standard x-ray films don't show it. Athletes who sustain this difficulty usually experience knee pain behind and to the outer border of the knee, and there will be varying degrees of knee instability. Reconstructive therapy does away with this problem.

Posterior cruciate ligament injury is caused by either a fall on the knee with the ankle in forced plantar flexion or a blow to the front of the tibia. In contrast to an anterior cruciate ligament injury, this trauma may not force the athlete to stop competing. However, he will have rear knee pain, dislocation of the tibia, and loss of the normal prominence of the tibial plateau beneath the femoral condyles. Reconstruction of this torn ligament by means of proliferant injections corrects the disorder.

Patellofemoral subluxation may go unrecognized by the trainer, the athlete, and even many doctors. A subluxation is a partial dislocation of a joint, so that the bone ends are misaligned but still in contact. Diagnosis of subluxation is difficult because the patella does not remain in a subluxated position and the patient shows minimal swelling and reports poorly localized, nondescript knee pain. As implied, an athlete may not report or even be aware of the transient malposition of the patella, because after injury he or she usually can continue competing and only experiences instability of the knee with sudden starts and stops and during cutting and agility drills. Reconstruction therapy corrects this patella problem, too.

Fibular head dislocation occurs because the athlete slips, suddenly inverting the ankle and forces it into plantar flexion, and falls on the leg with the knee flexed under the body. Sports in which this mechanism of injury is common include ice skating, baseball, soccer, and basketball. All athletes with this injury experience knee pain. Some have difficulty bearing weight and extending the knee and experience transient shooting pain down to the ankle or foot. However, many can walk with mild discomfort so they don't seek medical attention for weeks or months.[6]

Of course, at the risk of being repetitive, reconstructive therapy is the effective means of correcting fibular head dislocation. The vast majority of knee problems in sports or in everyday activities can be resolved with this treatment procedure.

Chapter Twelve
Reconstruction for Elbows, Ribs, Ankles, and Feet

Boyd C. Maxwell of Merced, California, thirty-eight years old and a stock broker, decided that he was not going to put up with the discomfort any longer. It was preventing him from concentrating on brokerage transactions. He was experiencing a cramping pain in the ulnar distribution of his left arm above and below the elbow and added numbness in the fourth and fifth fingers of that same limb. So, he walked into the office of neurologist Harish P. Porecha, M.D. of Modesto, California and asked for help. One of Maxwell's clients had told him that Dr. Porecha was the physician to see in that northern California city for musculoskeletal problems and sports injuries. On an emergency basis, Dr. Porecha fit the new patient into his crowded schedule because Maxwell came from a far distance and was in obvious pain. The broker explained that he is left-handed and found it impossible to write with the aching arm in its state of disrepair.

It seems that Maxwell hurt himself recreationally while working out as the proverbial weekend athlete. He plays squash with a passion but only on weekends, and it was after such a workout that his elbow hurt. He went to his local medical doctor, in Merced, who told him to go home and put on a heating pad, plus he prescribed the painkillers Tolectin™ and Tylenol with Codeine, #3™ for the patient. Within the week and because of his pain, Maxwell had consumed nine tablets of each medication. His stomach felt upset, and he still was disabled.

Upon examining the stockbroker, Dr. Porecha found, in addition to his left arm and hand problems, that he had tenderness over the cervical vertebrae C6 and C7. When his neck was moved Maxwell complained, as well, of pain in the pectoral regions of the left side of the chest near the coracoid process and the left deltoid muscle. Conduction of nerve impulses in the left ulnar nerve was normal.

It was apparent to the physician that someone with such a high- powered, type-A personality must play his squash games intensely and violently. The man admitted that he does play hard, fast, and without giving quarter.

His own left shoulder, back, arm, and hand symptoms could certainly be the consequences. Dr. Porecha's diagnosis turned out to be radiculopathy on the left side stemming from strain of the seventh or eight cervical vertebra and severe tearing of ligaments in the left elbow. As has been mentioned in other cases cited in this book, radiculopathy or radiculitis is inflammation of a nerve root, usually as it emerges from the spine. The condition, which invariably is disabling and painful, usually results from an injury — most suffered in automobile accidents, others in sports or from blows or falls. Less frequently, infections, growth or metabolic disorders may cause the nerve root inflammation. We had offered as a prior example of radiculopathy acute brachial radiculitis, which produces the shoulder girdle syndrome, evidenced by wasting of the shoulder girdle muscles and accompanied by sudden onset of acute pain in the shoulder which may radiate to the arm or neck.

While Maxwell exhibited these same sort of symptoms (but not shoulder muscle wasting), he had no evidence of any entrapment of the ulnar nerve at the elbow. In his September 1989 letter describing the patient's problem, Dr. Porecha states: "Even with physical therapy at our office, the man's elbow pain level on a scale of 0 to 10, was at 3 to 5. Because of that continuous near-mid-range pain, a series of proliferative injection treatments was begun on him. Two cubic centimeters (cc) of Lidocaine, 2.2 cc Colchicum, and 1.1 cc Pulsatilla [an herbal homeopathic remedy] was given into the left elbow. Immediately the patient's steady pain decreased to a minimum. He was able to move his arm readily. Within three days after the injection treatment he returned to unrestricted work writing with the left hand and using a data processor. I re-examined him about seven days later and found that he was doing well and needed no continuation of the injection series. Just the single set of injections was required to correct his sports-related injury.

"I sent Mr. Maxwell back to his original physician for continued care and thus familiarized another doctor in California with the benefits of reconstructive therapy," advised Dr. Porecha.

Anatomy of the Elbow Joint

The arm is jointed at its midsection by what is known as a "trochoginglymus," which means it is a compound joint or articulation consisting of a hinge and a pivot (see Figure 28). The semilunar notch of the ulna bone is hinged with the hyperboloid trochlea of the humerus bone. The proximal head of the radius pivots with the spherical capitulum of the humerus and also glides against both the proximal and distal ends of the ulna. The lower end of the humerus curves slightly forward, placing the articulating surface on top (dorsally). This shape places the normal position of the forearm in slight flexion, which increases the mechanical advantage of the arm's flexor muscles. The articular surface of the distal end of the humerus is cylindrical and smooth except for all but approximately 35 degrees of its circumference. The whole joint bends like a door hinge.

The trochlea is a pulley-shaped surface with depressions

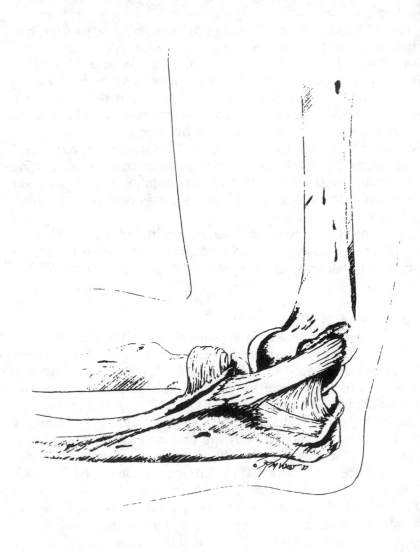

Figure 28. Ligaments of a normal elbow.

into the shaft of the humerus at both front and rear. The trochlea's front depression is the coronoid fossa which lodges the coronoid process of the ulna when the elbow is flexed. The rear depression is the olecranon fossa which lodges the olecranon process of the ulna when the elbow is extended. These fossi increase the range of motion of the ulna and allow a total excursion of about 140 degrees. The olecranon process restricts hyperextension of the elbow. The shape of trochlea and the closely fitting semilunar notch limit ulnohumeral movement with only an insignificant shift medially (toward the body) in flexion and laterally (away from the body) in extension. The trochlea and the capitulum are separated by the crest which fits into the notch between the ulna and the radius and serves as the bony guide of the elbow joint.

The concave head of the radius glides against the spherical surface at the capitulum of the humerus. The excursion of the head of the radius over the capitulum in full flexion is about 140 degrees. The rim of the head of the radius turns in the radial notch of the ulna, allowing a rotation of nearly 180 degrees. During pronation of the forearm the ulna remains fixed and the radius crosses over it. In supination the bones are uncrossed. The head of the radius is held in a tissue sling by strong collateral ligaments which stabilize this freely moving bone. The radius and ulna are bound together by an interosseus membrane which prevents an upward thrust of the radius and checks supination and forms a basis for insertion of the flexors and extensors of the deep muscles of the forearm.

In joint reconstruction, therapists are most concerned with the articular capsule and the ulnar collateral and radial collateral ligaments. The front and back parts of the capsule are broad and thin fibrous layers of connective tissue covering all surfaces of the joint. It is attached to the bony structures already described. The ulnar collateral ligament is thick, triangular and consists of two banded portions united by a thinner intermediate portion. These bands joint the humerus and ulna. The radial collateral ligament is a short and narrow fibrous band, less distinct than the ulnar collateral, attached, above, to a depression in the humerus, below to the annular ligament (which encircles the head of the radius and retains it in contact with the ulna.

Signs of Correction with Reconstructive Therapy

When tearings of the elbow ligaments take place, as occurred to Boyd Maxwell (see Figure 29), multiple injections in a set or series are given in and around these ligaments and their encompassing articular capsule. The reaction is exactly the same as happens in all other joints receiving reconstructive therapy.

James D. ZeBranek, D.O. of Garden City, Michigan, in a 1985 roundtable discussion of reconstructive therapy among members of the American Association of Orthopaedic Medicine explained that "sclerotherapy is a word coined back in the 1930's meaning production of scarification in the lumen of a blood vessel and, subsequently, then applied to mean the same thing in other tissues injected. We don't think that this is so [sometimes reconstructive therapy is referred to by long time users of the treatment as sclerotherapy] and the term is a misnomer."

A better term is joint reconstruction or joint healing or joint refurberation by natural means, Dr. ZeBranek suggested — thus eventually arriving at the best term: reconstruction therapy. "Going to the sclerosant solutions, these are generally graded, in my opinion," he continued, "much like when we use phenol coefficient in antiseptics. They are graded from the mildest sclerosants producing the least amount of artificial inflammatory activity to the greatest inflammatory producer to the least, which, in my opinion, is 25 percent dextrose."

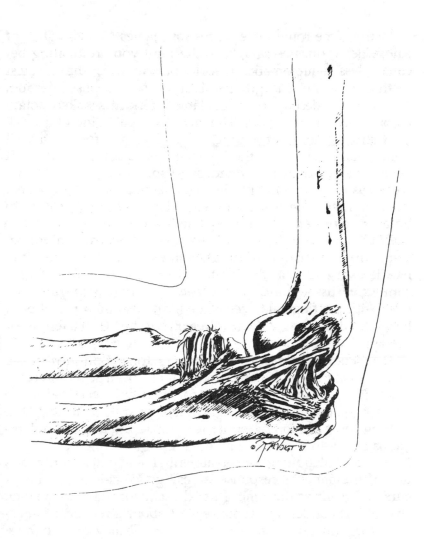

Figure 29. Torn, overly relaxed, and loosened ligaments of the elbow.

In the same roundtable discussion, James Carlson, D.O. of Knoxville, Tennessee said, ". . . the joint you are treating becomes less symptomatic. Needle palpation is the greatest method of evaluating [joint stability], pre and post injection. We liken the description to sticking a fork in a baked potato before and after it is done. The feel of the palpation of a weak or destroyed ligament is much like sticking a fork in a well done baked potato. As the ligament increases in strength, it takes on a feel of a raw potato, so to speak. Of course, from a spinal aspect, we can usually see the restoration of normal joint alignment once the joint capsules are strong enough to hold the joint in the correct position."

William Kubitschek, D.O. of San Marcos, California, responding to Dr. Carlson's remarks, added, "Using the needle as a gauge in the joint to determine buildup [of new connective tissue], and also physically using pressure sensation [with the fingers] to see if the joint has built up will both be good determining factors regarding the effectiveness of therapy."

Kent Pomeroy, M.D. of Phoenix, Arizona continued in the discussion of signs of correction with reconstructive therapy. Dr. Pomeroy said, "I'm looking for improved stability of the joints with manual testing and range of motion testing. I'm looking for reduction of tenderness where the tendons or ligaments attach to the bone. I'm looking for a retained correction after manipulation or self-treatment. I may inject only one time if the patient's response is very good. This probably occurs 5 percent of the time. I tell the patient that the average patient has the desired response after about three sets of injections for joint trouble of a minor nature. It may require more sets of injections to get the desired results and after the desired results are achieved, a booster injection may be required monthly or semi-annually. The patients' own healing responses, their tissue production, their state of health or nutrition, and their activities, determine how they will respond to [proliferating] injections."

At the conclusion of the administration of a skilled and trained physician's reconstructive therapeutic technique for a patient, the individual's joint, such as the elbow shown in Figure 30, has acquired new connective tissue. The new tissue is called cicatrix. If looked at under the microscope as in a biopsy, it will be seen that thicker fibers with more tensile strength than original normal ligaments are present (see the illustration of Figure 28).

A Veteran Reconstructive Therapist Speaks Out

V.A. Leopold, D.O. of Garden City, Kansas has practiced osteopathic medicine for 63 years and has incorporated reconstructive therapy as part of his treatment program for the musculoskeletal system. He declared himself in correspondence to us to be more interested in preventative medicine than just rendering corrective care. Dr. Leopold, coming from his broad experience, at age 92, having entered premedical training in 1921 and graduating from a college of osteopathic medicine in 1925, has set some standards for modern osteopathic and other medical doctors. He became a member of the College of Osteopathic Surgeons in 1937. He wrote, "I believe the medical profession in general has fallen down in learning and making a thorough study of preventative medicine. We certainly need more research in this area. I am very much interested in finding the cause of our patients' health problems, not just treating the symptoms instead of searching for the cause of the given condition at hand.

"There is always a cause for a health problem. It may be physical, structural, emotional, infectious, or even spiritual. I realize that medicine and surgery have made very good progress in many phases of health problems, but when you stop to really give it some thought we find that the structural

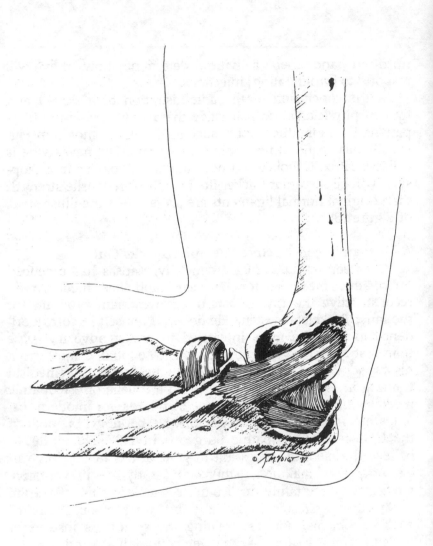

Figure 30. Stronger, firmer, reconstructed ligaments of the elbow. Torn and relaxed tendons (not pictured) can be reconstructed with the same method of reconstructive therapy.

part of the body is sadly neglected, even in the best medical hospitals. I am especially thinking of many minor deviations from normal, that definitely have their effect on the balance of the body. The orthopedic surgeons do some very fine work in fractures, disease of the bone, complete dislocations, protheses of hip joints and other joints, and are to be commended for their work," agreed Dr. Leopold. "I refer these types of cases to orthopedic surgeons. But now I am talking about the minor structural deviations from normal in the ribs and spine, including curvature, in which the condition should be referred to the physician who specializes in the structural portion of the body.

"We need mutual referrals to be made for the patient's best advantage and to save him or her pain, time, and money. Why accept a case of sciatic neuritis being sent to a hospital, for example, to be cared for there when, more than likely the hospital fails to have an osteopathic physician on the staff to correct the cause of pressure on the sciatic nerve, by correcting a fourth or fifth lumbar vertebral subluxaion or a sacroiliac joint that is out of place? I have seen these people lying in hospital beds with a bucks extensions attached [erroneously] for weeks, the hospital staff giving the patients morphine. Drugs are not good treatment for the sciatic nerve. This is a structural problem and requires corrective treatment [by means of manipulation with reconstructive therapy] to save the patient time, pain, and money," added Dr. Leopold. "This [drugging] process is absolutely 'pulling the wool over the patients' eyes' and should be changed. If we were honest with our patients, our liability insurance [costs] would be a lot lower. Patients wish to be treated as any physician would treat his own family members."

Reconstructive Therapy for Ribs and Shingles
Dr. Leopold went on to describe an unfortunate woman

near to his own advanced age who had difficulty with the viral disease shingles and associated subluxation of the rib cage. "An elderly lady in a wheelchair [Alice MacDonald of Dodge City, Kansas, age 89] with a broken hip that had never healed, partly because of diabetes, approached me in the nursing home in which she was spending her twilight years. I took care of several patients in this hospital-type facility, and I had taken care of her at different times during an earlier period. When she saw me, she burst out crying and asked if I could do anything to help her. Well, she was in this nursing home located near to Garden City under another doctor's care. I told her she would have to get permission from her own doctor to have me render any service.

"She asked him, and he immediately told her that if any doctor could help with the pain to go right ahead and get assistance. He had been applying soothing salves and other topical remedies for a couple of weeks but to no avail. Most physicians don't like to doctor a patient who has a condition which will not respond to their treatment," Dr. Leopold said, "and this woman had shingles (herpes zoster) around her rib cage."

Shingles usually starts with pain along the distribution of a nerve (often in the face, chest, or abdomen), followed by the development of vesicles. The disease subsides eventually, though sometimes severe pain may persist for many months in the area of the affected nerve. The virus that causes herpes zoster can also cause chickenpox in children.

Dr. Leopold continued, "She was very obese and with the fractured hip it was difficult to get her in the proper position to correct the rib lesion. Mrs. MacDonald was lying on the side of the problem rib facing the wall. I traced the shingles around the rib cage and found the displaced rib. I could almost hang my hat on it, it was so displaced.

"I injected an anesthetic with only a very slight amount of

sclerosing solution in the syringe [to furnish a minimal amount of reconstructive therapy]. I placed 5 cc of the solution in the facets surrounding the sixth dorsal vertebra and also the same amount at the head of the protruding sixth rib," he said of his procedure. "For fifteen minutes or so I visited with her until my anesthetic took hold. Then I placed both thumbs on the head of this displaced rib and in seconds it slipped out from under my thumbs and was corrected. The pain was absolutely gone immediately. And a few days later the shingles went away. I made a real friend in Alice Mac-Donald and impressed her physician, too.

"Remember this," admonished Dr. Leopold, "there is always a vertebral, rib, or sacroiliac problem present whenever shingles is on the scene. Why do these kinds of cases go for a year or two before finally healing on their own? Because most physicians don't recognize structural displacement as the true cause."

D.E. Imhoff, D.O., reconstructive therapist of Oregon, Ohio advises that he utilizes a proliferating solution composed of glucose, glycerin, and phenol for ligaments of the rib cage, lumbosacral, and sacroiliac areas. Dr. Imhoff usually achieves his objective with an average of three, four or five visits, during which time he injects the appropriate ligaments with his proliferant solution. Complex cases do require more treatment.

Instructions by Dr. Hudgins to his Joint Reconstruction Patients

Eighteen-year-old Kenneth Ferguson of Washington, D.C. had a workers' compensation claim as a result of injury on the job. He was a trainee in construction and hurt himself while lifting a heavy load of concrete. His chief complaint was pain in the mid- dorsal region of the back but especially around the ribs, mostly on his right side. Examination by F. Curtis

Hudgins, D.O. of Arlington, Virginia indicated to him that Kenneth had a serious rib lesion with somatic dysfunction of the lower and mid-dorsal thoracic region. Dr. Hudgins used reconstructive therapy for Kenneth's thoracic spine and rib cage. He gave weekly injections until the patient reported no more discomfort. In fact, the young man felt so well after receiving the first proliferating injection series that he lost no time from work at all.

Dr. Hudgins' instructions to his patients when he is administering reconstructive therapy are the following:

1. Always walk a little, perhaps a city block, after receiving your series of proliferant injections.

2. Do not apply heat such as a heating pad, don't take prolonged hot baths or hot showers after the injections.

3. If you take sacroiliac ligament reconstructive therapy, you will probably notice that you need about four, five, or six injection series before you have a finished result. Vertebral injections higher in the spine may respond faster.

4. If any allergic reaction such as a skin rash appears, please inform your reconstruction therapist.

5. If, after two days following your injection series, you feel any discomfort such as back pain or leg pain, you should return to the doctor for an examination and evaluation.

As an addition to Dr. Hudgins' suggestions, we wish to warn you away from consulting other physicians who are untrained in reconstructive therapy if some problem with the injections occurs. Since they don't understand the treatment procedure or how to cope with a possible complication, their ministrations will be ineffective or even detrimental to the joint reconstruction process.

One session of reconstructive therapy by Ellis V. Browning, M.D. of Yuma, Arizona solved the problem of a dog track announcer, fifty-six-year-old Irving Constantine, also of Yuma. Mr. Constantine had suffered with chronic, daily pain in the right lower ribs following a fall down stairs four years before. He had taken steroid injections, analgesics, bed rest, physiotherapy, chiropractic treatments, and muscle relaxants as the result of previous recommendations by doctors, relatives, neighbors, and friends, but nothing helped him.

Despite the track announcer's fear of injections, he had reached a point at which any kind of treatment was acceptable in order to be rid of his rib pain. Dr. Browning placed the proliferating solutions directly into the rib attachments of ligaments and tendons. The patient was free of pain right away and has remained so for over twelve years (to the present). This single session of reconstruction therapy is not the usual course of events for resolving years of pain and other symptoms. Yet, it does happen. More often a series of multiple injections is required for maximum benefit.

Reconstructive Therapy Alleviates Ankle Injuries

"I remember seeing this fifty-year-old white woman, Sarah Wanamaker of Redondo Beach, California, who related her tale of twenty-five years of chronic right ankle pain with swellings all around the ankle. She was unable to stand for any great length of time, and that's why she kept her job as a cashier in a busy restaurant," explained Joan M. Resk, D.O., J.D. of Huntington Beach, California. "It had her sitting down for the entire working day. She hated the job, Ms. Wanamaker told me, but it kept her off her feet so that the ankle didn't hurt.

"When Sarah consulted me a few years back, her right ankle was about twice the size of the left with marked swelling of the extremity below the knee," Dr. Resk explained. "She had visited about twenty-five different doctors in as many years. Quite frankly, I wondered, 'What can I do to help this patient after all that time and that huge number of physicians who had failed to assuage her problem?'

"Well, I checked over the area and found a marked instability of the right ankle. I told the patient what I had discovered and that, in essence, without a sound ankle or foundation to stand upon there was no way I could add anything more that the twenty- five other doctors had done. I then suggested that we might try reconstructive therapy, and the patient picked up on my words," said Dr. Resk. "She had me detail every aspect of the injection procedure. With her consent, I proceeded to use the basic reconstructive therapy solution of dextrose, Carbocaine, and Calphosan to inject into this patient's ankle.

"I did a series of seven injections comprising three individual injections per visit. At the end of that time the patient was verily elated. The swelling was gone; her right ankle was now of normal size; the pain had disappeared; the patient's limb was no longer weak because strength had returned to her ankle once again. Reconstructive therapy had done for Sarah Wanamaker what so many years of various other medical opinions and treatments had not done. It made this patient functional and free of pain," concluded Dr. Resk. "I heard from her a month later that she had quit her job as a cashier and had become a tour guide at a museum in Los Angeles."

Anatomy of the Ankle

The lower leg resembles the forearm in that it is composed of two long, thin bones, but, because of the leg's weight-bearing function, that's where the resemblance ends. The tibia, the heavy major weight-supporting bone of the lower leg, is enlarged at each end to form the articulation at the upper end with the femur and at the lower end with the talus of the foot. The fibula is the other long, thin bone which articulates with the tibia, but does not articulate with the femur or the patella. It does not form any portion of the knee joint. The lower end of the fibula creates part of the outer edge of the bony saddle that rides astride the talus bone.

The fibula, in addition to forming the outer aspect of the ankle joint, also acts as a weight-supporting strut. Its ends provide bases for attachments of some of the tendons in the heavy leg muscles. The end of the tibia at the medial malleolus is grooved for the passage of the large tendons in the foot. These bands support the arch of the foot as well as flex the toes and act in the extension of the ankle.

Any slight side-to-side motion of the ankle joint is allowed only by a stretching of the ligaments binding the fibula to the talus and by a slight bending of the shaft of the fibula. The fibula is readily broken when a large lateral force is applied to the ankle. When the fibula breaks, the total weight of the body is then shifted to the medial malleolus of the tibia and if the force is great enough, the tibia is also broken.

The superior articular surface of the talus is wedge-shaped with the front part broader than the back. In dorsiflexion the talus wedge spreads the lateral and medial malleolus apart. The stress is taken up by a slight rotation and bending of the fibula and a slight stretching of the ligaments uniting the bones of the ankle. If a force is applied to the back of the leg while the ankle is dorsiflexed, the action of the wedged talus will be to shear the medial and lateral malleoli. The ligaments, especially the deltoid ligament binding the tibia to the talus and the calcaneus (the heel bone) as shown in Figure 31, are so strong that they can resist a force which will fracture the bones to which they are attached. This type of injury occurs when a person slips and falls upon his foot when it is tucked up under him.

Most of the time when ankle twisting takes place, of course, these strong bones do not break but rather the ligaments tear or become overly stretched and relax (see Figure 32). Sprained or strained ankle is the result with its typical state of inflammation. The ligaments involved in such inflam-

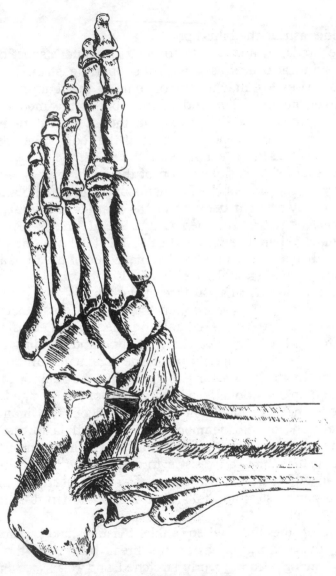

Figure 31. The stabilizing ligaments of a normal ankle. (Forefoot tendons and ligaments are not shown.)

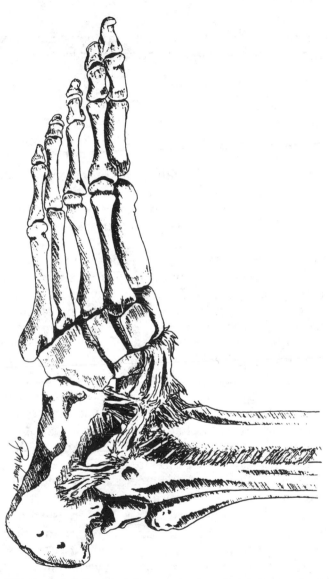

Figure 32. Torn and loosened ligaments of a chronically sprained unstable, weakened ankle. Tendons (not shown) may be strained and weakened as well.

mation typically are the deltoid, talonavicular, posterior talofibular, calcaneofibular, and lateral talocalcaneal.

Chronically Strained Ankle Ligaments Corrected

In 1958, Gordon J. Bronston, D.P.M. of Chicago submitted a paper to the American Podiatry Association (APA) on "The Strengthening of Chronically Strained Ankle Ligaments with Injections of Sodium Psylliate" to the William J. Stickel Annual Awards for Research in Podiatry. Dr. Bronston's paper won Honorable Mention from the awards committee.[1]

Dr. Bronston's paper was an exceedingly important piece of research writing and deserved greater recognition than it received. Dr. Bronston wrote:

> Chronic strain and laxity in the ligamentous structure of the ankle underlie many of the orthopedic problems related to this articulation. This paper presents a new method of approach for the treatment of these conditons. Though this research has been concerned primarily with the ankle, the basic principle of strengthening and shortening weak and lax ligaments can theoretically be applied to any podiatric problem wherein these structures are involved. . . . Chemically, sodium psylliate is a mixture of the sodium salts of five fatty acids: oleic, linoleic, linolenic, palmitic, and stearic, placing it in the same chemical category as the soaps. The final product is a mixture of a 5 percent solution of sodium psylliate and 2 percent benzyl alcohol. When this product is injected into a ligament it acts as an irritant to the fibroblasts of the ligament starting an inflammatory reaction. Within five days the fibroblasts can be seen in the tissue. Within two weeks new bundles of dense fibers appear. By the eighteenth day most of the fibrous tissue appears mature, although it takes approximately six weeks until the process is com-

pleted.

The results of injection as described in this paper by Dr. Bronston may be seen in Figure 33. Just as he explains, new ligamentous tissue has been laid down as regrowth or new growth of connective tissue fibers from the fibroblasts.

Dr. Bronston went on to describe the safety of sodium psyllate injections. He then pointed out the conditions which respond to treatment with this proliferating agent. He wrote:

> Since any weak or lax ligament can be strengthened and/or shortened, theoretically any ligamentous problem involving a chronic sprain or joint instability due to a lax or elongated ligament could be corrected. With regards to the ankle, the most common of these problems is the lateral ankle sprain with the resultant lateral instability. The patient who is constantly turning over on the affected ankle, especially while running or engaged in some sport, or the person who complains of pain and edema [swelling] in the lateral ankle area are common examples of this type of involvement. . . .

Then, for the edification of his podiatric colleagues who might be intrigued enough to attempt reconstructive therapy for their own patients, Dr. Bronston added:

> It is advisable not to use an extremely fine gauge needle because one important guide to accurate injections is the resistance offered the needle by the fibers. Too fine a needle could pass between these fibers and go completely through the ligament without an awareness of this, thereby losing the effectiveness of that injection. . . . The first treatment usually consists of only one injection in order to observe the patient's reactions, if any. Following this, any number of injections can be given although the maximum number necessary per visit usually does not exceed four. The length of time between treatments will vary from five to ten days. Week-

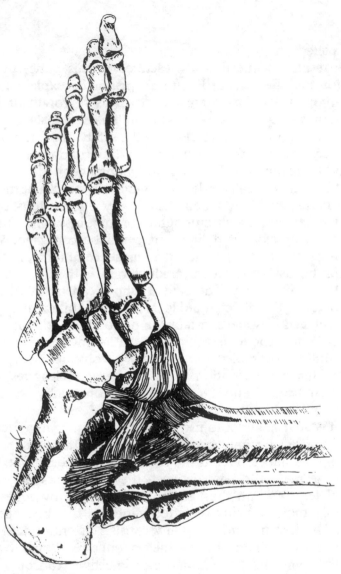

Figure 33. Permanently reconstructed ligaments that are stronger and firmer allow the ankle to function normally. Tendons (not shown) may also be reconstructed.

ly injections are usually sufficient, however. . . . The overall period of treatment lasts approximately six weeks. Although the average number of injections per ligament is three or four, supportive therapy should be continued for at least a six-week period to insure a good result.[2]

Reconstructive Therapy Is Useful for Foot Joints

Little Johnnie Quigley, age nine, of Grand Island, Nebraska had a hard time running, jumping, playing baseball or performing the other activites boys his age ordinarily do. His legs seemed not to function as well. He was always the last one picked for a team when the kids chose up sides to play a game. In truth, the lad was suffering psychological effects from his physical inferiority, and he manifested emotional difficulties too.

His mother, Margaret Quigley, took Johnnie to visit an orthopedic surgeon when the physical education teacher at grade school alerted her that something was wrong with the child's legs. The orthopedist said that his achilles tendons were floppy and weak. The Quigleys had a choice. Either Johnnie must refrain from any vigorous physical activity or he could have an operation in which his achilles tendons would be surgically shortened and then put into plaster-of-Paris casts for two months. While recuperating, he would have to use a wheelchair. Upon removal of the casts, he would need another five or six months of physical therapy to rehabilitate his muscles so that he might learn to walk again.

Mrs. Quigley was shocked by such drastic measures for her little Johnnie. Consequently, she took time to check around and learn where else treatment for her son's condition might be found. The mother and son traveled to Fullerton, Nebraska for consultation with Arthur Dowell, M.D., a reconstructive therapist. After examining the boy, Dr. Dowell told the mother about the injection technique using proliferating solutions. He believed that the procedure probably would correct the boy's overly elongated and lax achilles tendons. In fact, Dr. Dowell had taken Dr. Faber's preceptorship program in reconstructive therapy, so that he was well prepared to help little Johnnie. The mother agreed to have this treatment for her son.

Just one week after the child had received a single series of injections into both sets of tendons, it became obvious to Mrs. Quigley that reconstructive therapy was making a big difference. Within a month of weekly treatments, the physical education teacher telephoned to say that he noticed Johnnie was much more athletic. The teacher wanted to know about the course of treatment being followed so that it might be recommended to other parents for their children. He was amazed, the teacher said, because Johnnie was running and jumping with the best of them.

The injection series actually produced the desired shortening of the boy's achilles tendons, and no surgical procedure was ever required.

Chapter Thirteen

Treatment of Hip Trouble, Associated Sciatica, and Carpal Tunnel Syndrome of the Wrist

At age 69, Fred Shull, M.D. of Bellingham, Washington had been providing gynecological and obstetrical service to the women of his community for over forty years. Now his friends counciled him to go into retirement. "It's time to enjoy the 'golden years,'" they said. "Join us on the golf course or come along for a climb up the mountainside."

Dr. Shull decided that his buddies were offering good advice, so he hung up his scalpel and stethoscope in favor of the leisure activities he had always missed. It wasn't golf and hiking that he loved so much as the more unique hobbies of roller skating and artistic kite flying. After turning over his patient files to other physicians and closing his office, he attempted to fulfill his dream of spending days at leisure. Roller skating at the rink and running to catch the wind with his kites were out of the question, however, because for years a gnawing pain in his left hip had been steadily increasing. He walked with a limp in order to take pressure off the painful hip joint. It was a deep, penetrating ache that was always with him, and there were overtones of sciatica running down the leg from his left posterior sacroiliac region.

The largest nerve in the body, the sciatic nerve — two of them — one running down each leg — begins at the lower spine and goes down the thigh to the knee, where it divides

217

into two main branches that give rise to a complex network of nerves supplying the lower leg and the foot. Measuring 4/5 of an inch in breadth, it is a continuation of the sacral plexus inside the pelvis and passes out through a bony opening to the back of the thigh. There it divides into two branches to supply the leg and foot. It may give rise to sciatic neuritis (to be described in a later section in this chapter) some of which Fred Shull was experiencing.

The radiologist at Bellingham General Hospital took radiographs of Dr. Shull's pelvic region and pointed out the severe degeneration easily seen throughout his left hip joint. The x-ray expert asked, "Fred do you know that you need to have a hip replacement procedure? Why don't you see our staff orthopedic surgeon for implanting an artificial hip prosthesis? He'll have you installed with a new hip in no time!"

As it happened, around the time Dr. Shull sought medical attention for his left hip, the *Journal of the American Medical Association* reported in its July 10, 1987 issue, "More than 126,000 hip replacement procedures are performed annually in this country and, because of the 'graying of America,' that number is likely to increase. But orthopedic surgeons are concerned by reports that too many — the number varies with surgical series being reported — artificial hips become loose and need to be surgically revised."[1]

It turns out that the human body, including the hip, often rejects joint attachments with artificial materials. Such substitutes for natural tissues as "baling wire, sealing wax, chewing gum" or other additives to body parts — cemented hip implants included — are destined for eventual failure.

William H. Harris, M.D., chief of the Hip and Implant Unit at Massachusetts General Hospital, Boston, cautions that most replaced hips fail because of stress over a period of years. In a study presented at the American Academy of Orthopaedic Surgeons annual meeting, one surgical team indicated that 24 percent of patients in the teams' operated groups were rated as "unsatisfactory" eight years after undergoing their hip surgeries.

Having graduated from Princeton, Yale, and the State University of New York at Buffalo, and having been an obstetrical and gynecological surgeon, Dr. Shull was no stranger to the art and science of surgery. He knew that all operations potentially were dangerous. In his practice, he had tried to avoid surgery for his patients at all costs. He learned that the body heals itself most of the time without medical invasion. The physician and surgeon can best help a patient by avoiding drugs and surgery. "Do everything possible to optimize healing," was his philosophy. The human body is smarter than high-tech artificial medicine will ever be. "Dr. Fred," as he was called by his patients, believed each person's soma (body) is truly miraculous.

So, he was in a dilemma. Fred Shull, M.D. understood that he had to take action, since his hip pain was growing worse day-by-day. Hip surgery was not his area of expertise, but he instinctively knew: "as God makes little green apples, hip surgery was not for me."

One day in February 1987, while reading *Health Freedom News*, the journal of the National Health Federation, a nationwide organization dedicated to the preservation and restoration of your right to determine your own health care, an article caught his eye. It was titled, "Permanent Stabilization of Tendons, Ligaments and Joints," by William J. Faber, D.O. Dr. Shull recognized that this might be the alternative he was looking for — a form of biological or "complementary" medicine that could solve his hip trouble.

After telephoning Dr. Faber, Dr. Shull flew to Milwaukee for a musculoskeletal evaluation and possible treatment. He carried his pelvic x-ray films with him. Physical examination, case history, and radiographic review all having been conducted, the Milwaukee osteopathic physician told the Bellingham medical doctor that reconstructive therapy could very well accomplish the hip restoration. Dr. Shull responded, "Let's do it."

Dr. Faber gave him aggressive therapy, administering four sets of proliferating injections in that single week. He told the patient to go back to Bellingham and telephone when he noticed a change in his hip joint. Dr. Shull called one week later, saying, "I can feel the strength in my hip increasing daily. All kinds of good things have happened. I can walk well, climb stairs, get out of chairs, and even fly my kites while running into the wind. It's amazing! I'm going to try roller skating next. This correction is a lot easier than I thought possible."

"Congratulations, Fred, your body has a healing ability and is saying a strong 'Yes' to reconstructive therapy," replied Dr. Faber. "You merely have to repeat the therapy until maximum strengthening occurs. Let me give you the address of another reconstructive therapist located closer to you." For followup, Dr. Shull was referred to Richard Koch, D.O. of Olympia, Washington, a skilled therapist in joint reconstruction.

This former practicing gynecologist received the additional joint reconstruction procedures from Dr. Koch and experienced continued improvement. Dr. Shull reported to us recently that he roller skates several times a week and belongs to a roller skaters' club. He does his indoor skating when he's not out jogging through Bellingham's streets, hiking Washington State's mountain trails, golfing its eighteen-hole courses, or kite flying in the open countryside. He performs any type of sports activity he wants without a second thought to his once-impaired left hip. It's not degenerated anymore inasmuch as new connective tissue growth has filled in around the ligaments supporting the hip articulation.

Anatomy of the Hip Joint

The articulation between the head of the femur and the acetabulum (cavity) of the hip bone is a ball and socket joint. This hip joint permits movements of flexion, extension, abduction, adduction, circumduction, medial rotation, and lateral rotation of the leg. The limit to which dancers, high jumpers, and high hurdlers can elevate and spread the legs is determined by the flexibility of the ligaments and muscles, not by the arrangement of the bones of the hip joint.

Extending from a pit in the central portion of the head of the femur to the margin of the acetabular notch, and probably assisting in holding this large joint together, the ligamentum teres lies within the joint cavity (see Figure 34). For the most part the integrity of the hip is maintained by the pressure of the atmosphere against the partial vacuum within the joint. A capsular ligament completes the fastening of the head of the femur to the acetabulum of the hip bone.

The capsular ligament has three thickenings named the iliofemoral, ischiocapsular, and pubocapsular ligaments. The iliofemoral ligament resembles an inverted Y and is attached above to the ilium and below to the intertrochanteric line of the femur. The ischiocapsular ligament passes from the ischium into the capsule. The iliofemoral and ischiocapsular ligaments increase the stability of the hip joint in the standing position. The pubocapsular ligament passes from the pubic bone into the capsule and prevents excessive abduction of the femur. The combined capsular ligament is so strong that a dislocation is less common than a fracture of the bones of the hip.

Certainly the hip's ligaments can strain, sprain, laxate, and tear. As indicated in Figure 35, if this hip joint trauma continues over a prolonged period, osteoarthritis also may be the result. The joint degenerates and forms solid bubbles of excess mineralization with calcium salts derived from the blood

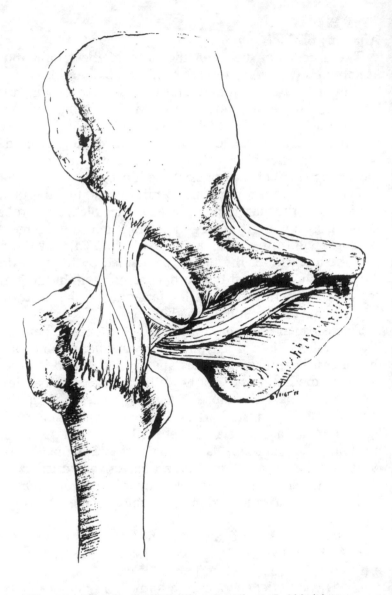

Figure 34. The large stabilizing ligaments of a normal hip joint.

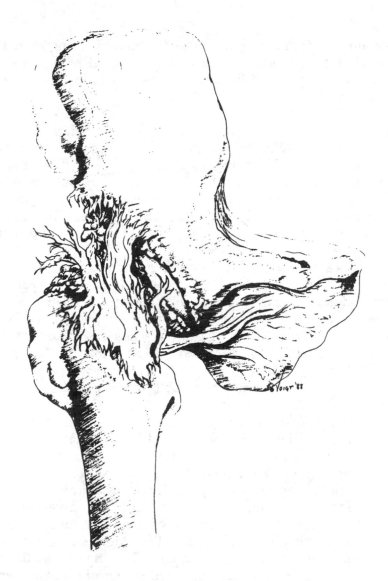

Figure 35. Torn, loosened, and weakened ligaments that are producing an arthritic hip joint where metastatic calcium is laid down.

stream. Calcium being the most voluminous mineral in the blood — required for a host of physiological processes — it deposits at the site of ligament looseness within the hip joint in a metastatic form.

How Torn Pelvic Ligaments Cause Associate Sciatica

We have previously described sciatic neuritis, often called sciatica, as an inflammation of the sciatic nerve. It is a gnawing pain usually felt in the back of the thigh and down the legs, descending from the buttocks and frequently accompanied by numbness in the region of the ankle. When due to spinal root involvement, it is aggravated by change of posture, coughing, sneezing, or defecation.

Sciatica has many causes, however, and aggravation is easily given to bring on the shooting, burning pain. For example, constipation or sitting on a cold bench may cause sciatic neuritis of short duration, soon relieved by a laxative or warmth. The real source of chronic sciatica is sometimes difficult to determine. One major cause described by George S. Hackett, M.D. and T.C. Huang, Ph.D. is sciatica-type pain as a complication of posterior sacroiliac ligament relaxation.[2] They wrote:

> Barrages of sensory and antidromic impulses induced by traction-stimulation on non-stretchable sensory nerve fibrils within the fibro-osseous attachment of weak sacroiliac ligament fibers are the cause of pain and neurovascular dystrophy (decalcification) of the sacrum and ilium [and hip joint]. The decalcification weakens the attachments of the sacrotuberous and sacrospinous ligaments and the tendons of the piriformis muscle, so that they become the origin of additional barrages of impulses that overwhelm the sciatic nerve components resulting in the production of pain, inflammation, dystrophy, and dysfunction. It is a vicious circle

224

of ligament relaxation and decalcification in which either may induce the other. The diagnosis of ligament relaxation is by trigger-point tenderness. It is invariably confirmed by intraligamentous needling with local anesthetic solution.

The effective treatment for sciatica involving hip degeneration recommended by Drs. Hackett and Huang consisted of reconstructive therapy to permanently strengthen the ligament attachments with new bone and fibrous-tissue cells to stabilize the sacroiliac joint (see Figure 36) and eliminate the pain, including sciatica. This is the very treatment that aided Fred Shull, M.D.

Dislocated Hip Prosthesis Corrected
with Reconstructive Therapy

Harold C. Walmer, D.O. of Elizabethtown, Pennsylvania reported on a 67-year-old woman, Rhonda Marshall, whose locomotion was severely limited because of a progressive osteoarthritis of the right hip. In November 1978, she underwent an operation for a total hip replacement, using the Sbarbaro Total Hip Prosthesis. Two weeks following surgery, while moving in her hospital bed, Mrs. Marshall dislocated her hip. Reduction and correction was carried out the following day under general anesthesia. On December 28, 1978, the patient was hospitalized with phlebitis of the left leg. While a bedpan was being placed under her, the patient dislocated her surgical right hip for the second time.

In May 1979, while she was bending forward to pull a weed from the garden, the hip dislocated again. With professional help, Mrs. Marshall had it put back in place. Subsequent dislocations occurred on July 10, 1980, July 15, 1980, and January 10, 1981. All of these dislocations occurred while the patient moved in bed. All but one of the dislocations required emergency room hospitalization to reset the hip in

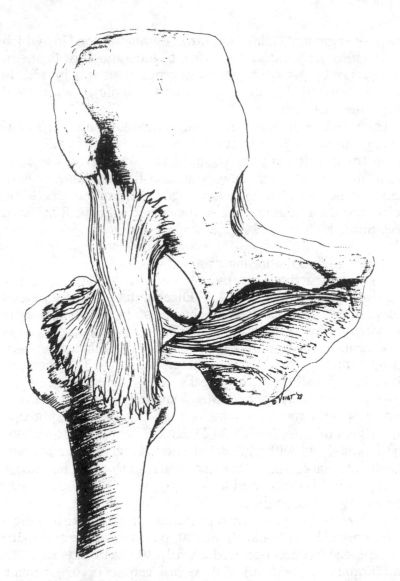

Figure 36. Permanently reconstructed ligaments that are stronger and firmer, allowing the hip joint to function normally.

place. Four surgeons explained to the patient that once a hip dislocates, the capsular ligaments become severely stretched and each dislocation then encourages the next one. Mrs. Marshall was not anxious to have her artificial hip replaced surgically however.

It was then, in April 1981, that this homemaker traveled from Olean, New York and presented herself at the Elizabethtown, Pennsylvania office of Dr. Harold Walmer. It's not unusual for patients to travel long distances to seek out the services of the few American physicians who are skilled in reconstructive therapy. The trip was worth it, Mrs. Marshall reported to Pennsylvania physicians interested in her case. First she told what it was like to undergo the hip operation and then experience its after-effects.

She said, "Since having my hip surgery, I have never been able to walk any distance or stand for any length of time without pain. Sitting down for even a short period of five to ten minutes helps to get going again. It seems that the longer I allow the pain to persist, the longer it takes to eliminate it later."[3]

Reporting on the procedural technique of his treatment for permanently correcting a dislocated hip prosthesis to his state osteopathic colleagues, Dr. Walmer wrote that proliferant injections were given to Mrs. Marshall on April 13th and 21st, May 5th and 19th, and June 9th and 30th. "There was moderate postinjection pain for several days after each treatment," he said. The results were gratifying for both patient and doctor. He further wrote:

By June 9 the patient reported that she could stand longer than previously. On June 30, 1981, the patient reported that her hip felt stronger and had very little pain and that she could walk longer without experiencing pain. By September, 1981, the patient had no pain in her hip. On October 13, 1981 she reported that she was walking better than she had in many years. By February 1, 1982, the patient was walking in snow on uneven terrain with no pain. On February 7, she fell on ice directly on the involved hip, sustaining a bruise but experiencing no dislocation. There have been no dislocations since sclerotherapy [reconstructive therapy] was instituted.

While traditional methods of treatment for degenerated hips include the routine placement of metal screws, metal rods, and artificial joints into hips, these operative procedures fail to provide patients with any lasting comfort. The recipients of such techniques usually suffer from complications such as an overweight condition, long durations of illness, severe arthritic disease, and multiple major surgeries. Yet, frequently as their last resort these people have benefited greatly from applications of reconstructive therapy.

Reconstructive Therapy for Wrist Trauma

From the East Texas town of Henderson, a rodeo rider named Jerry Masap, 29 years old, sustained an injury eight years before when he fell from a bronco during a wild west show. This left him with pain in his right wrist with even the slightest activity. He was certain that his failure to become rich and famous on the rodeo circuit was directly due to the disability in his right hand. He had to make do with his left hand, although he had been born right-handed

It was a long time in coming, but finally Jerry found his way to John L. Sessions, D.O., physician and surgeon in the Jasper County Medical Center of Kirbyville, Texas. After conducting the usual examination procedures and determining the cowboy's source of trouble, Dr. Sessions administered reconstructive therapy to his right wrist. "Jerry improved with the first proliferant injection into the wrist," Dr. Sessions said in his May 22, 1989 letter. "He was 90 percent better after receiving seven injections. He is still under treatment, and I expect total recovery."

During the eight years he was doctoring, Jerry Masap had tried many other medical specialists who had applied splints, casts, diathermy, cortisone injections, cortisone pills, exercises, other drugs and pain-killing medicines. None of these had any significant effect, but reconstructive therapy provided him with recovery within a few weeks. When the authors checked with Dr. Sessions about the cowboy's recovery, we learned that altogether nine reconstructive treatments had been required to give him complete comfort and correction of his wrist problem. He is now winning big prize money as a bronco buster and calf roper. Jerry was able to renew an old skill — throwing a lariat accurately — because he had use of both of his wrists and hands once again.

Anatomy of the Wrist

The normal wrist (see Figure 37) has seven bones, the trapezium, trapezoid, capitate, hamate, navicular, lunate, and triangular, arranged in a half shell formation in such a way that the midposition of the hand when freely extended is about 12 degrees in hyperextension and three degrees in abduction. During abduction of the hand the navicular and the trapezium are spread since they are not tied together to any great extent by ligaments. During adduction the carpal surfaces become more tightly compressed. The carpal-metacarpal articulation of the fingers is amply fortified by a ligamentous apparatus which covers the joints in all directions.

The wrist joint is a condyloid articulation. The parts forming it are the distal end of the radius and under surface of the articular disk above, and the bones of the wrist below. They form a transversely elliptical concave surface. The joint is surrounded by a capsule and strengthened by the following ligaments: the volar radiocarpal, the dorsal radiocarpal, the ulnar collateral, and the radial collateral. The volar radiocarpal ligament is a broad membranous band, attached to the radius and

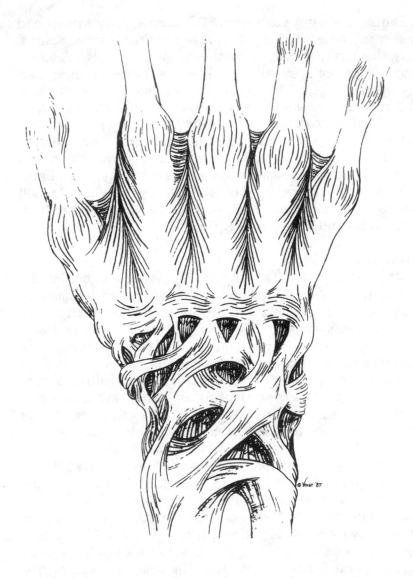

Figure 37. Top of the hand showing the normal ligaments of the wrist.

the ulna; its fibers pass downward to be inserted into the navicular, lunate, and triangular bones. The dorsal radiocarpal ligament is less thick and strong than the volar and extends fibers to the same bones. The ulnar collateral ligament is a rounded cord, attached to the ulna and to the pisiform and transverse carpal ligaments. The radial collateral ligament extends from the radius to some of the wrist bones.

When there is injury to the wrist with ligamentous lengthening and tearing, these more major tissues may be involved but also a variety of other sets of ligamentous structures are traumatized (see Figure 38). The connective tissues injured would be the two dorsal ligaments, the two volar ligaments, the two narrow bundles of interosseous ligaments, the articular capsule, and the synovial membrane. Injury may result from immediate wrenching, twisting, and crushing or, more commonly, from repeated micro- or mini-traumas related to motions performed using the same internal connective tissue structures over and over again throughout the day (such as assembly line work). Such repeated microtraumas may give rise to a condition that is growing in frequency among the populations of Western industrialized nations. The condition is known as carpal tunnel syndrome of the wrist. Modern industrial crafts, such as those activities involved in assembling, welding, and soldering for small appliance making or computer manufacturing, are the source of this wrist disability.

Carpal Tunnel Syndrome of the Wrist

A compression of the median nerve in the wrist as it enters the palm of the hand through the carpal tunnel gives rise to the chronic pain condition — carpal tunnel syndrome. The carpal tunnel is an existing space between the wrist's carpal bones and the connective tissue over the flexor tendons. Through the space pass the flexor tendons and the median nerve. When the median nerve is compressed, pain and

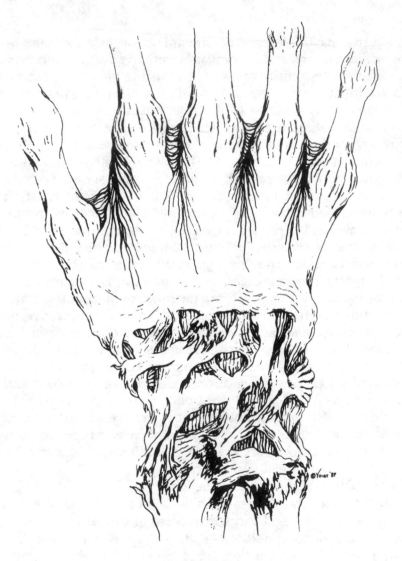

Figure 38. The top of the hand showing torn and loosened wrist ligaments from injury or from repeated actions of firm grasping and usage such as in assembly-line work.

numbness in the index and middle fingers and weakness of the abductor muscle of the thumb result.

Often therapeutic methods for carpal tunnel syndrome prove inadequate. The patient's night pain and difficulty in holding light objects are recurrent. Numbness, tingling, deep pain, and swelling are descriptive of what happens to the many who suffer with and find no relief for symptoms of carpal tunnel syndrome.

Extensive involvement of many nerves in the wrist and arm may simulate a polyneuropathy. Neuropathy is a symptom complex — a syndrome — rather than a disease. It is a syndrome of sensory, motor, reflex, and vasomotor symptoms, singly or in combination, produced by disease or microtrauma of a single nerve, two or more nerves in separate areas, or many nerves simultaneously. In carpal tunnel syndrome, the median nerve gets compressed between the longitudinal tendons that serve the wrist and hand muscles and the transverse superficial carpal ligament in the volar aspect of the wrist.

As suggested, carpal tunnel syndrome is diagnosed with increased frequency as more workers are required to perform repeated hand and wrist activities. Over 5,700 cases were reported in Wisconsin alone in 1987, according to worker compensation statistics. Many of these workers take medications, steroid injections, physical therapy, and undergo surgery without achieving satisfactory results. There is one treatment that works remarkably well, however (see Figure 39). Of course, it is reconstructive therapy. This restores fibrous growth to the affected ligaments and so strengthens the traumatized wrist that it becomes more facile even than when it was normal.

Diagnosing Carpal Tunnel Syndrome

Although well-described in the medical literature, carpal tunnel syndrome may be difficult to diagnose because it gets

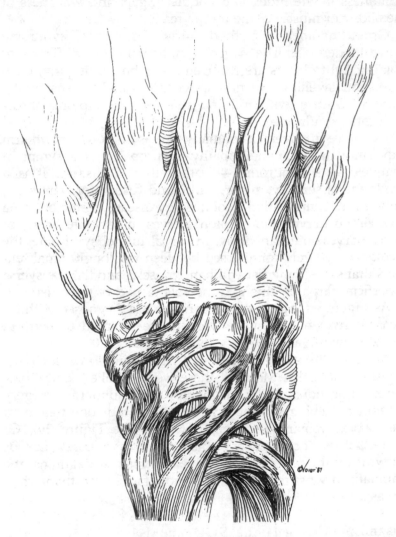

Figure 39. Formerly damaged wrist ligaments restabilized, strengthened, and functioning normally from reconstructive therapy.

confused with wrist instability, a concept totally overlooked in medical- surgical diagnosis. The carpal tunnel syndrome has been considered a chronic disease with a fixed set of symptoms, affecting women between the ages of 40 and 60 years. There may be a combination of neck and wrist pain, especially in people with osteoarthritis. Hand numbness may be present, associated with proximal extension of pain to the forearm and occasionally to the arm, shoulder, or even up to the ear. Older patients sometimes claim that their fingers are stiff when, in reality, they are numb.

Ligaments and tendons are very tough and strong. When they become damaged they tend to become torn where the ligament or tendon attaches to bone. First there is swelling on the back of the wrist. The swollen areas are distant from the bones that encase the carpal tunnel and also distant from the transverse carpal ligament on the palmar side of the hand and wrist. Pain is usually located over the radiocarpal ligament on the thumb side of the wrist, over the ulnarcarpal ligament near the small finger-side of the wrist, and on the edges of other carpal bones on the top of the wrist. All of these areas are quite remote from the carpal tunnel.

Another indicator of ligament or tendon weakness is lack of grasp strength. Patients often report that they drop items when doing aggressive activities and that they tend to fatigue easily. Dr. Faber's testing of these patients reveals that they often have only 20 percent normal strength. Ligaments and tendons play a major role in a person's strength for grasping, but nerve damage can also cause weakness and this fact complicates diagnoses.

In severe cases, indicators of weak wrist ligaments rather than carpal tunnel syndrome are clicking, popping or grinding in the joints. This can be detected in less overt phases by putting the individual's wrist through its range of motion while placing the examiner's palm over the back of the patient's wrist. Any slight popping, snapping or grinding shows that there is weakness and instability of the ligaments and tendons involved. Wrist motion should be smooth and free from any crepitation.

An individual with carpal tunnel syndrome and a person with ligament weakness and instability in the wrist can be helped by bracing. The brace takes the place of normal ligaments. When choosing a brace the type that supports the entire wrist should be selected and not just a wrist strap. A proper wrist brace also has metal support which extends into the palm. Velcro straps help the brace to fit snugly. Digits should be free to move and the brace should be worn for entire days, because most victims have severe pain at night.[4]

Many conditions can mimic the carpal tunnel syndrome, but the patient's medical history and the doctor's physical examination of him or her often miss the real cause, because the art and ideas in this book are not yet appreciated by the vast majority of practicing clinicians and surgeons. Robert J. Spinner, M.D., John W. Bachman, M.D., and Peter C. Amadio, M.D. from the Mayo Medical School offer a number of conditions associated with the problem including rheumatoid arthritis, systemic lupus erythematosus, scleroderma, polymyalgia rheumatica, eosinophilic fasciitis, gout, degenerative arthritis, nonspecific tenosynovitis, trigger finger, Dupuytren's contractor, Paget's disease, diabetes mellitus, obesity, pregnancy, tumors, and at least a dozen more. These are swelling conditions of metabolic imbalances causing carpal tunnel syndrome. By far, however, repetitive movements and grasping are the most frequently attributed reasons.[5]

The Pianist's Overuse Syndrome

As an illustration of this repetitive movement problem, a computer program developed by Purdue University researchers shows pianists how they may be able to alleviate hand pain by changing the position of their fingers at the piano. Pianists sometimes suffer from a form of carpal tunnel syndrome designated as "overuse syndrome." Ben M. Hillberry, professor of mechanical engineering at Purdue, and graduate student David C. Harding created the computer program that sheds light on the hand pain. They say the research, which could eventually help people in other hand-intensive occupations, provides an alternative to pianists to cutting down on playing hours, the traditional treatment for the pain.

Information released in a special report from Purdue University on September 14, 1989 indicates that while physicians have no difficulty diagnosing the common syndrome, in the past they often could not explain its exact cause or why one pianist would suffer from it while another would not.

Pianists were chosen for study because their finger movement is primarily two-dimensional, although the research likely is applicable to players of string and wind instruments, engineer Hillberry says. Hillberry and Harding used a special piano that they calibrated to record the force of a finger's impact on a piano key. At the same time, video cameras record from the side and from above the exact angle of the finger on the piano key. When these data are entered into the computer program, the program can calculate the forces at each of the finger joints and tendons for the subject's playing style.

The most harmful way to play the piano, it turns out, is to play with straight or nearly straight fingers parallel to the keyboard. Bringing the fingers into a more curved position alleviates joint stress.

Carpal Tunnel Syndrome Completely Corrected

Any process that encroaches on the median nerve within the carpal tunnel, either extrinsically or intrinsically, can lead to carpal tunnel syndrome. Repetitive motion, overuse, vibration, and direct trauma have been described as possible industrial causes of carpal tunnel syndrome.[6] The same sort of torn and loosened wrist ligaments occurring from acute and sudden injury, as shown in Figure 38, can show up from repeated actions of firm grasping and usage such as in assembly-line work. However, formerly damaged wrist ligaments may be restabilized, strengthened, and made to function normally by employing reconstructive therapy. The actual increase in the injured ligament or tendon can be greater than 100 percent (as illustrated in Figure 39).

This was the case for Miriam Fascia of Davenport, Iowa, age 43, who is employed as an assembly line production worker in a mill that makes pillows, quilts, comforters, and feather beddings. She was the victim of carpal tunnel syndrome. "I am more than 100 percent improved over what had been my wrist problem," Mrs. Fascia said. "For three years I couldn't wear any rings because of the swelling into my fingers. My wrists constantly hurt me terribly. I kept losing hand strength and the ability to conduct a normal life. For example, I couldn't pick up a toothbrush to clean my teeth. I couldn't comb my hair. Opening a car door was impossible. I had to ask strangers to do it for me. I was unable to lift a cup of tea without feeling pain run up either of my wrists along the back sides. I wasn't able to open a jar of pickles. My wrist muscles felt like they were perpetually overstrained, although I know now it was not a muscle involvement but rather my ligaments were too relaxed.

"I had wrist braces made, but wearing them prevented me from working. So I removed them during the time at work and suffered absolute agony. Most times I worked double shifts, too — sixteen hours — because my family needs the money. My husband takes special treatment for his MS. I swallowed tons of aspirin so that I could sleep. I figured that if I was allowed to sleep, I could live with the pain at work the next day," explained Mrs. Fascia. "It got to me after a while."

First treated by one of the most skilled, gentle, and well-loved chiropractors in the midwest, Jarka Odvarko, D.C. of Bettendorf, Iowa (one of the Quad Cities along the Mississippi River), Mrs. Fascia is the sole support of her spouse of 22 years, who has suffered with multiple sclerosis during their entire married life, and of her four children. Repeated complaints by the patient of constant pain in both wrists moved Dr. Odvarko to refer her to Dr. Faber specifically to receive reconstructive therapy. "It was a God-send to me that she did that," said Mrs. Fascia. "I still go to Dr. Odvarko once a month, because she is working with Dr. Faber to keep me in tiptop condition, but the reconstructive therapy has given me comfort that I've not known for years. I've continued to work double shifts which got me promoted to tougher, more skilled work at a higher rate of pay now that my carpal tunnel syndrome is solved."

Examination by Dr. Faber indicated to him that Mrs. Fascia's carpal tunnel syndrome would respond well to the proliferative injection procedure. She accepted treatment and found that her crepitus (grinding noise), night pain, swelling, and pronounced loss of the ability to grasp steadily got better. "Driving four hours each way to get my wrist joint reconstruction was the best investment in time and money that I ever made," said the patient.

She noticed that she sounded (as Mrs. Fascia described it) "less like a bowl of Rice Krispies with my wrists snapping, cracking and popping." Instructed by previous physicians to wear hand traction braces at all times, after a series of just five proliferating treatments she was able to discard the two braces. Then with seven injection series completed she was transferred to a more vigorous job demanding greater ability with her wrists and hands.

"At one time, before I met Dr. Odvarko and found hope and comfort through her ministrations, the University physicians told me I'd just have to live with the pain or undergo surgery," said the woman. "But you better believe that when she referred me to Dr. Faber a whole new world opened for me. The reconstructive treatment gave me a reason to be happy with living once again. My wrist pains went away after the first two injections, and they have never come back. For the optimum wrist endurance that reconstructive therapy allows, I've taken more injections as a kind of insurance against getting carpal tunnel syndrome again. My hands and wrists are better than ever before."

Her employer was gratified by her therapeutic results because five more of his quilting workers have Mrs. Fascia's same problem. If those workers respond well to the same treatment, it could markedly cut down on his factory's Workers' Compensation insurance premiums. He has now sent his other employees with carpal tunnel syndrome to receive reconstructive therapy in Milwaukee.

As stated in the institution's July 1989 issue of it's journal, The Mayo Clinic realizes that surgery for carpal tunnel is often unsuccessful in dynamic use carpal tunnel syndrome. In particular, The Mayo Clinic says, this lack of success occurs if the patient returns to the same environment of repetitive wrist and grasping motions.

In summary, the authors concur that carpal tunnel syndrome is most often misdiagnosed. Cutting stabilizing ligaments cannot make a wrist stronger. The swelling in the wrist and its "carpal tunnel" is secondary to stretched and torn ligaments and tendons that cause instability, weakness, pain, numbness, and other difficulties. Reconstructive therapy provides unsurpassed results for dynamic carpal tunnel syndrome.

Coauthor Dr. William J. Faber anticipates studying further and publishing research on reconstructive therapy. Giving such research on chronic joint pain exposure in professional journals and consumer magazines will help people avoid destructive surgery. The United States will be able to compete more effectively in the world economy if this country's work force can remain healthy and free from chronic joint disabilities.

Chapter Fourteen

Manipulation in Combination with Reconstructive Therapy

In the spring of 1983, Tommy Lourie was twelve years old. He had red hair, a happy nature, and an abiding love for soccer. The boy had played since he was only six years old and showed talent. He lived in Brussels, Belgium where his father, a member of the U.S. Navy, was stationed. Toward the end of the school year Tommy began to complain of vague back pain. It hurt to tie his shoes and to kick the soccer ball. His parents thought it was "growing pains" (even though it doesn't hurt to grow). Nothing was done therapeutically to reduce the boy's discomfort. When the school term was over, Tommy flew to San Diego to visit his paternal grandparents for the summer.

Almost immediately upon seeing him, his grandmother noticed that Tommy seemed to be twisted. He did not walk erect. His left shoulder blade seemed to "stick out," as she described it. Grandma Lourie made arrangements for her grandson to see Andrew L. Kulik, D.O. of San Diego. This osteopathic physician specializes in structural evaluation, manipulative therapy, and reconstructive therapy. Standing in shorts with his back to the physician, the patient was observed to have a pronounced scoliotic curve — the spine curved like an "S". One hip was higher than the other causing the scapula (shoulder blade) to protrude markedly, just as Grandma Lourie said.

242

On structural examination while the lad was lying in the prone position, his two internal tibial (lower leg bone) malleoli were compared and found to be at different levels. Tommy's hip bones were not even either. His spinous processes in the back from the sacrum to the occiput followed a typical scoliotic pattern with muscle rigidity throughout the entire spine. Palpation by Dr. Kulik of the patient's sacroiliac ligaments revealed pain on pressure on the right side. Since the signs pointed Dr. Kulik toward the diagnosis of a right sacroiliac malpositioning, he decided to do a standard manipulative maneuver on the boy. Reconstructive therapy, the doctor judged, was unnecessary. He moved Tommy's right ileum on the sacrum by having the patient lie on his left side, underarm back, and body twisted so as to lock the lumbar vertebrae. The doctor placed his one hand over the upper sacroiliac joint and with the other hand under the patient's upper bent knee joint, he lifted the leg, carried it in a semicircle toward the boy's head, then brought it down to complete extension. The strong adductor muscles pulled the pelvis backward against the counter force of the other hand. The doctor felt a definite rotary movement under his hand and heard a heavy "thump" as the joint moved to its normal position.

Following this, he asked Tommy to stand and walk around. There was no trace of scoliosis. Dr. Kulik's examination of body landmark levels showed all to be even. By this simple one-shot osteopathic maneuver, Tommy Lourie was cured of his scoliotic curvature and relieved of his discomfort, possibly forever.

The boy returned to Belgium and spent the winter playing soccer. After the school term he returned to his grandmother's home in San Diego where he was re-evaluated by Dr. Kulik again. There was no sign of abnormal spinal curves. Landmarks in the prone and supine positions showed no change — all were normal. In addition his musculature was much improved. Now, nearly seven years later, his sacroiliac has not slipped at all. His spine has healed very well merely from the single osteopathic manipulative correction.

Joint Manipulation as Therapy

Manipulation or the repositioning of the structural anatomy of bones, tendons, ligaments, disks, and cartilage is probably the most effective single method of treatment administered by osteopathic physicians and progressive-minded allopathic physicians for the more common musculoskeletal problems. Chiropractors make very effective use of manipulative techniques, as well, although they have their own methods of movement.

Osteopathic manipulation treats musculoskeletal dysfunction that mimics or aggravates symptoms of organic disease. It aims to restore full range and quality of motion to joints affected by muscle spasm, swelling, and fibrosis. Fibrosis is the thickening or scarring of connective tissue, most often a consequence of inflammation or injury. Where bony fusion or osteophytes (spurring) limit range of motion irremediably, osteopathic manipulation aims to help the patient compensate.[1]

However, "Osteopathic manipulative therapy is a much misunderstood clinical tool," said Edward G. Stiles, D.O., a general osteopathic practitioner in Norman, Oklahoma and associate clinical professor, biomechanics department, Michigan State University, College of Osteopathic Medicine, East Lansing. Dr. Stiles instructed a group of allopathic physicians, including physiatrists (specialists in physical medicine), during a mini- course on osteopathic manipulation sponsored by *Patient Care* magazine.

As Dr. Stiles described it, the misunderstanding of osteopathic manipulation occurs, in part because of the ways some practitioners describe it. "Manipulative therapy does not

244

involve 'putting things back into place,' as some have said,"
he explained. "Nor does it cure conditions such as migraine or
angina pectoris, as a few practitioners have claimed.

"With manipulative therapy we can treat pathologic alteration in the motion of joints — what has come to be called
somatic dysfunction. This mechanical dysfunction of the
framework of the body — the soma, or musculoskeletal system — can be associated in various ways with organic disease:
it can mimic disease; it can aggravate the symptoms and signs
of existing disease; it may often be a result of the body's attempts to cope with disease. Consequently, while manipulation won't cure angina or pleurisy, for instance, it can clear up
somatic dysfunction of the anterior chest wall that may
produce symptoms easily mistaken for those of angina or
pleurisy," said Dr. Stiles.

"The motion of any joint is normally restricted by anatomic
barriers — limits beyond which any movement will result in
dislocation or fracture. Just within the anatomic barriers are
so-called physiologic barriers — limits determined by muscles,
tendons, and other soft tissues in the area. The joint can be
moved beyond these barriers to the anatomic barriers outside
them, but some external force is normally required. For instance, if you ask someone with normal range of motion to
turn his head as far as possible to the right, he or she will be
able to reach the physiologic barrier; but if you hold the head
in that position for a moment, allowing the muscles to relax,
you can turn the head a little farther to the right by applying
a small additional force," Dr. Stiles continued. "By so doing,
you can take it up against the anatomic barrier. In general, the
active range of motion of a joint is defined by its physiologic
barriers, and its passive range of motion is defined by its
anatomic barriers.

"When I say that manipulation treats pathologic alteration
in the range of motion of a joint, I'm referring to conditions

that limit active movement of the joint to less than the full range defined by the physiologic barriers. A patient may have a vertebra, for example, that rotates left up to the physiologic barrier but is stopped short of the physiologic barrier when it rotates right: It encounters a pathologic barrier," he said.

"A pathologic barrier may result from any of a number of conditions, of course, including pain, muscle spasm, edema, fibrosis, osteophytes, and surgical fusion of a joint. To treat the dysfunction of a joint properly, you need to establish the nature of the pathologic barrier," Dr. Stiles said, "which you can usually do through careful palpation and motion testing of the joint."

Then Dr. Stiles described some simple diagnostic factors to the physicians listening:

- "Pain is easy enough to identify. The patient says, 'Ow! That hurts,' as you reach the pathologic barrier.
- "If the barrier is due to muscle spasm, you'll be able to feel a sudden localized spasm as the joint reaches its pathologic barrier.
- "Edema resulting from an acute injury can cause soft tissues surrounding the joint to feel boggy, swollen, and congested as you reach the barrier.
- "If the barrier is a chronic condition, there will probably be fibrosis in the area of the joint when you get to the pathologic barrier and motion stops, you'll feel a little give; you'll be able to spring the joint a bit, but you'll feel that you're fighting some resistance — that you're stretching scar tissue.
- "If the barrier is due to osteophytic changes or, say, to spinal fusion, the barrier will feel hard; you won't be able to spring the joint beyond it. And in the case of surgical fusion, of course, you will be able to see the identifying scar," concluded Dr. Stiles.[2]

Three Types of Manipulation

Thus, manipulative therapy involves the operator — usually an osteopathic, chiropractic, or allopathic physician — handling soft tissues in order to achieve healing by means of muscle relaxation. Such muscle relaxation is done by putting a joint through its range of movement to increase that active range of movement. If the joint is painful, it should be supported so that mechanical stresses on overly relaxed or torn and inflamed ligaments — the main source of pain — are minimized. This demands skill on the part of the manipulator. The ultimate phase of most types of manipulative therapy is corrective, applied by a deliberate thrust or jerk to increase joint mobility, taking the movement a bit farther than it goes in ordinary active movement but within the normal passive range. There may be some momentary discomfort for the patient who is not under anesthesia (anesthesia is hardly ever used), but the process usually has no pain connected with it.

There are a few systems of manipulative technique, and each manipulator has his own favorite set of methods. It is practically impossible to make objective comparisons of different methods. The judgments about success or failure of the methods are strictly subjective.

Dr. Stiles explained that there are three broad types of manipulative therapy: (1) muscle energy techniques; (2) a high- velocity, low-amplitude (HVLA) thrusting method; and (3) functional techniques. The muscle energy manipulation employs the patient's own muscle effort to restore the range of motion of a dysfunctional joint. The HVLA thrusting relies on force applied by the practitioner. Functional techniques require only gentle movement and careful positioning of the joint to reduce muscle tension and increase range of motion. All three methods are quite valuable therapeutically and comfortable in their application, but in unskilled hands HVLA thrusting is the most dangerous of the three. Dr. Faber prefers the gentler techniques of muscle energy manipulation and functional application to relax pathologic barriers to motion. These methods do not overstretch or tear ligaments, tendons or joint capsules.

Rene Caillet, M.D., Director of Rehabilitation Services Santa Monica Hospital Medical Center in Santa Monica, California, suggests that during manipulation, the muscle should be stretched as far as it can be, then given a further stretch as a thrust. When the muscles are stretched, both the long fibers and the spindle fibers are stretched. The thrust further stretches the spindle, which releases the spasm. Movement of the functional unit returns.

Dr. Caillet adds, "That the muscle spindle spasm is released by manipulation is purely hypothetical but appears feasible, as it is based upon the same principle as is stretch by exercise or by traction."[3]

Dr. Caillet believes that the reason manipulation decreases spasm and unlocks the joints of the spine and other restricted articular areas may be its effect on the joints' capsules. He correctly states that every synovial joint of the body must have a capsule surrounding it. This capsule contains joint lubricating fluid and cartilage that coats each opposing bone surface to form the articulation. "The capsule is thin, reasonably elastic, and waterproof, that is, it does not leak out the fluid. . . . Joint capsules are supplied with different types of nerves. Type I and Type II nerves act reflexly by going to the spine from the capsule, then connecting to other nerves in the cord to return to the muscles in the same vicinity of that specific joint. They theoretically can either relax or contract these muscles. Type III nerves from the capsule carry the sensation of pain."

Injury to the joint may have irritated the capsule and thus irritated the Type I and II nerves, resulting in spasm. Manipulation may interrupt this cycle by stretching the capsule, which, in turn, causes the muscles to relax. Accordingly, manipulation becomes an adjunct to reconstructive therapy.

When manipulation is applied in conjunction with proliferating injections the result will be quick relief of muscle spasm and the almost immediate return to movement. Without reconstructive therapy, however, manipulation is insufficient to prevent the return of spasm and joint irritation with chronic pain if tears or laxity of structures are present. The capsule tissues remain torn and inflamed and thus remain susceptible to a return of the protective spasm.

Although Dr. Caillet prefers exercise, proper alignment and training for joints to reconstructive therapy he says, "Repeated manipulations are to be condemned if they are not accompanied by the entire treatment program."[4]

Some Dangers or Contra-indications to Manipulations

The type of manipulation most osteopathic physicians have been taught over the years and the one most used by practitioners in general — osteopathic, chiropractic, and allopathic physicians, physical therapists, and some massage therapists — is HVLA thrusting. This high-velocity, low-amplitude thrusting involves positioning the patient so as to bring the restricted segment directly up against its pathologic barrier. HVLA manipulation differs from the more gentle muscle energy technique or the even gentler functional manipulation used at the Milwaukee Pain Clinic and Metabolic Research Center in that the force in HVLA used to alter the barrier is supplied by the practitioner rather than by the patient. The force is applied in the form of a carefully directed, sharp, short thrust.

Properly performed, HVLA techniques require very little force. Unfortunately, though, the amount of force used seems often to be inversely proportional to the understanding and skill of the clinician. Therefore, the dangers of HVLA manipulation come from people who know the least about it.

They are most likely to use excessive force and apply it improperly. These forceful practitioners get joints to pop, but those popping joints may be the wrong ones. They may produce too much motion in segments above or below the dysfunction site, helping the patient to compensate but leaving the original problem untreated. And if the practitioner produces high-velocity movement with a high amplitude, he or she may cause permanent damage.

According to Walter J. Treanor, M.D., associate clinical professor, department of medicine, University of Nevada School of Medicine, Reno, "Perhaps the most valid criticism of manipulative treatment is the oft-accompanying neglect of a basic diagnosis, particularly in underlying neurologic, orthopedic, and psychological diseases. . . . The three most important elements in the treatment of any disease are a correct diagnosis, a correct diagnosis, and a correct diagnosis."

Then Dr. Treanor suggested, "If manipulative therapy is ever to take an honored place in the medical armamentarium, it must satisfy the same rigid requirements of any other form of validated treatment:

- It must be proven in its efficacy over the long term.
- Its results must be reproducible by the skeptical.
- It must do no harm.
- Its advocates must temper enthusiasm with doubt."

Anthony G. Chila, D.O., professor and chairman, department of family medicine, chief of clinical research, Ohio University College of Osteopathic Medicine, Athens, agrees that diagnosis is imperative. Dr. Chila said, "Careful diagnosis by palpation is fundamental to the appropriate use of manipulation. Whether in examining the motion of a vertebral unit or in analyzing the character of soft tissues, sense awareness enhances diagnostic effectiveness. Direct sensory information is often more important than the information provided by conventional adjunctive laboratory and radiologic studies. The history and physical examination, corroborated by appropriate adjunctive studies and palpatory evaluation, form the basis for effective differential diagnosis."

"Though theory may differ as to cause or even effect, all practitioners of manipulation recognize that manipulation is indicated only when some 'barrier' to the normal motion of a synovial joint restricts this motion, usually only in one or two planes of the normal motion of that joint, and that there is an associated alteration of the 'end feel' or 'joint play,' which is the range between the extreme of voluntary or physiologic motion of a joint and the extreme of anatomic motion," said Stephen M. Levin, M.D., Secretary of the North American Academy of Manipulative Medicine and lecturer at the Michigan State University College of Osteopathic Medicine in East Lansing. "The joint play may be the only motion lost in a dysfunctional joint. All manipulative procedures aim to break down that barrier and restore joint play. Testing the barrier immediately after treatment provides instant feedback to the clinician as to his or her diagnostic and therapeutic skills."

The Recommended Form of Manipulation

Muscle energy manipulation or non-thrust methods are the recommended forms of manipulation when used in combination with reconstructive therapy. To perform effective muscle energy or non-thrust manipulation, you need to start with a precise structural diagnosis.

The first step in effective manipulation is always to carry out careful motion testing to determine which joints are restricted in which of their motions. It's not enough merely to localize the patient's problem to the lumbar spine, for instance; if the problem is that the left-hand facets of the fourth and fifth lumbar vertebrae don't open on flexion, the practitioner must know it. Working from the more general diagnosis, the doctor would not be able to position the patient so as to direct the proper force specifically to the restricted segment. He might free up the lumbar area without correcting the problem — by encouraging hypermobility in neighboring segments rather than normal mobility in the restricted segment.

Once the diagnosis has been made, the practitioner needs to position the patient accurately, so that his or her muscle effort concentrates force on the segment in question with pinpoint accuracy and applies the force in exactly the direction needed to counter the restriction.

Not much force is required with muscle energy or nonthrust manipulation. If the patient does what the practitioner directs him to do, everything will go fine. Sometimes a patient tends to confuse the reasons for the manipulation, thinking of it as a test of strength. Then he or she will injure the part being manipulated.

The medical consumer can try muscle energy manipulation on his or her own to see how it works. Do the maneuver to increase the range of internal rotation (toward the body) of the forearm in a friend. Test your subject's forearms to identify the one that has less range of motion. Then ask the subject to try momentarily to rotate the restricted forearm externally (away from the body) while you hold it firmly against the barrier limiting internal rotation. When he or she relaxes, you should then be able to internally rotate the forearm, without forcing it, past the original pathologic barrier.

Summarizing the Concepts of Manipulation

Manipulation of the musculoskeletal system by chiropractors, osteopaths, medical doctors, and other skilled technicians is a viable and proven technique for many hands-on diagnoses and treatments. It is most useful as a precursor technique applied before reconstructive therapy. Often, such joint, tendon, ligament, and bone manipulation can provide an alternative to more intrusive toxic therapies involving drugs and/or surgery.

Most osteopathic physicians utilize all of the recognized procedures and modern technologies for prevention, diagnosis, and treatment of disease, including nutrition, imagery, drugs, radiation, and surgery. But the D.O. also has another pair of tools that enable him or her to accurately diagnose areas of dysfunction and treat them effectively. These tools are the professional's hands.

Manipulation brings an added dimension to the therapist's diagnostic and therapeutic armamentarium. Sometimes it is in the form of palpation (touch) as a diagnostic procedure to detect soft tissue changes or structural asymmetries. Other times it is in the form of corrective thrust forces to relieve dysfunction or restrictions of motion in joints. Because musculoskeletal dysfunction can mimic other disease syndromes, manipulation is an important component in differential diagnosis, as well as a means of correcting structural problems.

It has been well-documented that diseases of specific organs can produce pain in distant parts of the body. Stomach ulcers consistently cause areas of spinal pain and irritation just below the shoulders in the back. The radiation of pain to the loin from a diseased kidney is another typical example, as is the reflection of pain and disability to the left shoulder following heart disease. In diagnosing such diseases, doctors using manipulation recognize that symptoms can be produced in healthy organs to which pain has been referred.

Conversely, disturbances affecting the musculoskeletal system can cause symptoms that simulate other illnesses. Among the most common causes of recurrent headaches, as we have cited, are disorders of the cervical portion of the spinal column. Consequently, properly applied manipulative treatment, particularly directed to the neck and head before the administration of reconstructive therapy, often affords relief of headache symptoms when all other remedies have failed.

The Full Spectrum of Manipulations

We have described only three — a small sample — of the half-dozen manipulation techniques that focus on the principal that body structure and function are dependent on one another. When structure is altered via the musculoskeletal system, abnormalities occur in other body systems. This, in turn, can produce restriction of motion, tenderness, tissue changes, and asymmetry.

Following are the full spectrum of the manipulation procedures used by practitioners like osteopathic physicians to diagnose and treat somatic dysfunctions:

Hands-on contact

The value of the placing of hands on a patient is universally acknowledged by health professionals as a functional stimulator. This essential component of the doctor-patient relationship has a great deal to do with the patient's well-being, whether he or she suffers from a cold or a terminal disease. When the D.O., D.C., N.D., or M.D. examines a patient by auscultation of the chest or palpation of the abdomen or spine, the treatment already has begun.

Soft-tissue Technique

This functional procedure is commonly applied to the musculature surrounding the spine, and consists of a rhythmic linear stretching, deep pressure, and traction. Its purpose is to move tissue fluids and to relax hypertonic muscles and myofascial (fibrous tissue) layers associated with somatic dysfunction.

Lymphatic Technique

This second functional method promotes circulation of the lymphatic fluids and can be used to relieve upper and lower respiratory infections. Pressure is applied with the physician's hands to the prone patient's upper anterior chest wall. When the force applied to the chest reaches its maximum on expiration, the physician's hands are removed suddenly. This action increases negative pressure of the chest to assist the body's respiratory mechanism to move lymphatic fluids.

HVLA Thrust Technique

In this previously described form of manipulation, the physician applies a high-velocity/low-amplitude thrust to restore motion to a joint. With such a technique, the joint regains its normal range of motion and breaks abnormal neural reflexes. The procedure reduces and/or completely nullifies the signs of tissue changes, asymmetry, restriction of motion, and tenderness associated with somatic dysfunction.

Muscle Energy Technique

Here, as we have discussed, the patient is directed to use his or her muscles from a precise position and a specific direction against a counterforce applied by the physician. The purpose is to mobilize a particular somatic dysfunction.

Counter-strain

With the counter-strain technique, the patient is moved passively away from the restricted motion barrier, toward planes of easy motion, searching for the position of greatest comfort. At this point, passive, asymptomatic strain is induced. This technique is indicated for relief of somatic dysfunctions that are too acute or too delicate to treat in other ways.

If you want to learn more about manipulation, contact any

of the following institutions. They can supply information about written materials, tutorials, and seminars available to help practitioners develop basic skills of osteopathic manipulation or to provide the layperson with a better understanding of the concepts. Contact the public relations departments of:

- American Academy of Osteopathy
  12 West Locust Street, P.O. Box 750
  Newark, Ohio 43055 — (614) 349-8701

- Michigan State University College
  of Osteopathic Medicine
  A-306 East Fee Hall
  East Lansing, Michigan 48824 — (517) 353-9714

- North American Academy of Manipulative Medicine
  5021 Seminary Road
  Alexandria, Virginia 22311 — (703) 931-0233

- Department of General and Family Practice
  Oklahoma College of Osteopathic Medicine
  1111 West 17th Street
  Tulsa, Oklahoma 74107 — (918) 582-1972

- Department of Osteopathic Principles and Practice
  Philadelphia College of Osteopathic Medicine
  4150 City Avenue
  Philadelphia, Pennsylvania 19131 — (215) 581-6430

- The American Osteopathic Association
  142 East Ontario Street
  Chicago, Illinois 60611 — (312) 280-5854

Manipulative therapy performed by osteopathic physcians, chiropractors, physiatrists, and other professional therapists expert in this technique has been praised for its remedial value. Many people have testified to the health benefits they've received from its use. Yet we wish to caution against letting manual manipulation become any kind of substitute for proper medical attention. In other words, don't let manipulative therapy become a replacement for competent medical advice.

Nothing written in *Pain, Pain Go Away* should be construed as prescribing therapeutically for any health problem. We do believe our recommendations are excellent procedures that will aid the user in the prevention and/or correction of disease, however, and toward this end we heartily suggest employment of reconstructive therapy. We make this recommendation especially if manipulation or other therapeutic methods fail to resolve pain and restore function.

Chapter Fifteen

'Hopeless' Cases that Found Correction with Reconstructive Therapy

An actively practicing "old-time family physician" in Lauderdale-by-the-Sea, Florida, Wilfred W. Mittlestadt, D.O., represents the best of Medicine's service to humanity. As he renders care to people in need, Dr. Mittlestadt explains to his patients about their ailments and suggests home remedies that could offer them relief or cure. He is friendly, concerned, compassionate, and comforting to be around. In administering therapy he deals with the entire person and not just his or her individual body part. Dr. Mittlestadt is a holistic physician.

Today, at age 83, after recently recovering from a cerebral vascular accident (a stroke), his overall health is good. But Dr. Mittlestadt's, musculoskeletal system was not always in good shape. When he was 19 and a telephone lineman for the county utility near his home in Fall Creek, Wisconsin, he was content to earn a modest living. This serenity was interrupted by an accident that seriously injured his spine. In a high wind on a rainy day, he was thrown from a telephone pole. The fall crushed eight of his midback and lumbar vertebrae. They were crumbled and brought on paralysis from the chest down.

Specialists judged that he was finished. They thought he would remain paralyzed and have to learn to live with pain, disabled for life in a wheelchair. This was over sixty years ago.

"At the time, attending doctors told me it was permanent,

that I'd never walk again," said Dr. Mittlestadt. "All except one osteopathic physician, that was Dr. Murphy, and I'll never forget him, for he had faith in the possibility of some recovery, if I worked with him toward this goal. He looked at me sharply, and I guess my eyes told him I would try, and he said, 'You will walk again.' It was like a promise I had to keep. So we worked together. I was in a body cast for six months in the hospital, and the night before the cast was removed, I had a vision in which I was assured I would keep the promise."

The osteopath worked diligently with his skilled hands to heal Bill's battered structure. With the aid of manipulative therapy, mobility slowly returned to his lower limbs, and he regained control of his bladder. The former telephone lineman was unable to walk very far, but he did walk. And he couldn't stand up straight, because he developed a four-inch deviation from normal as a result of his crushed vertebrae. These deviations, known as wedged compression fractures, caused him to remain in a definite and permanently set scoliosis pattern. He maintained a bent-to- the-side posture all of the time. His clothes had to be altered to accommodate the imbalances created by this scoliotic curvature (see Figure 40, a photograph of Dr. Mittlestadt's spine).

Young Bill Mittlestadt, with more specialized osteopathic assistance and continued rehabilitative therapy was not confined to a wheelchair as predicted by the medical specialists, but became ambulatory and eager to make his mark in the world. He decided to emulate the osteopathic physician who had faith in his recovery. He knew the man to be kind, remarkably adept with his hands, and a healer. So, young Bill recovered steadily to the point that he sought admission to professional school.

Dr. Mittlestadt became an osteopathic physician himself upon completing his training at the Chicago College of Osteopathic Medicine and Surgery in 1934. He practiced at

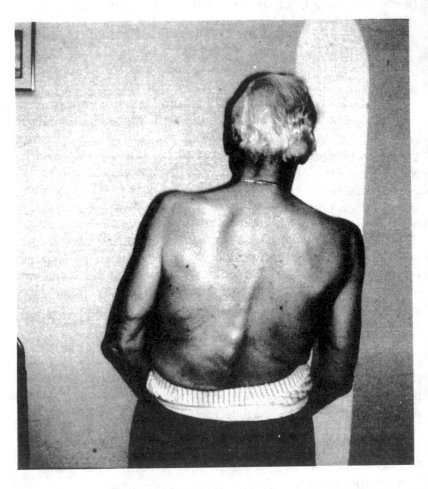

Figure 40. A photograph showing the scoliotic curvature of Dr. W.W. Mittelstadt. He attributes his recover from paralysis and multiple compression fractures 60 years ago to manipulation and reconstructive therapy.

Stevens Point, Wisconsin until 1938, when he moved to Marshfield. There he purchased and ran a 30-bed hospital, but he prepared for future semi-retirement by taking and passing the Florida State Board Examination in Osteopathy in 1963. In 1972, he made his final move to Lauderdale-by-the-Sea.

Dr. Bill Mittlestadt studied reconstructive therapy from medical pioneers George Stuart Hackett, M.D., E.H. Gedney, D.O., and David Shuman, D.O. The injection procedure helped him enormously to strengthen his spine and alleviate the chronic pain that shot up and down his back. At every seminar in which reconstructive therapy was demonstrated to fledgling therapists, Dr. Mittlestadt invariably was the human "guinea pig" volunteer who lent his back for treatment. He probably received a couple of hundred sets of injections, collectively totalling ten thousand needle sticks along his spine.

"My back got strong again," Dr. Mittlestadt exclaims. "Sure it's crooked as all heck, but it does okay by me. It stopped hurting years ago. I've been in continuous active practice using reconstructive therapy and biological medicine for my patients for over fifty years. I play 18 holes of golf with a usual score of 83." He makes sure to play the links at least three times a week, weather permitting, in sunny Florida.

Over the past forty years, Dr. Mittlestadt has received reconstructive therapy from possibly 150 colleagues who have practiced their techniques on his back. As many or more different types of proliferating solutions have gone into his connective tissues, which have added layer upon layer of needed structural support. While he's not been able to grow new bone to replace the crumbled vertebrae, his ligaments surrounding them have the tensile strength of steel. They allow him to walk without any pain or marked limp.

"I owe my life to osteopathic medicine and reconstructive therapy," says Dr. Mittlestadt. "Without them I'd surely would have had a hopeless life of being a cripple using wheelchairs and bed pans."

Jan Nissen, of Wausau, Wisconsin, by age 33, had undergone thirteen major operations on her left and right knees and three more surgeries on her hands because of completely destroyed rheumatoid joints. Two of the surgeries replaced her left joint knee bones with metallic substitutes, and the last procedure that she experienced took part of her abdominal muscle and used it to help stabilize the weakened knee. With all of the scars surrounding the joint, her knee looked like a road map. The total length of her scars in that one small area was over eight feet.

She had some of the country's foremost orthopedic, rheumatology, and neural specialists at leading medical centers caring for her, but to no avail. Rheumatoid arthritis was taking away her ability to function as a person.

The disease first struck her when she was just fifteen years old. By age 29, after her husband was killed in a train and car accident, the arthritis became highly aggressive, affecting her wrists, fingers, ankles, both knees, hips, elbows, shoulders, and neck. Perhaps it was the shock of her marital loss that brought on the rheumatoid flare-up. Nobody knows. But the symptoms and signs became overpowering for Jan, and she turned into a total invalid.

X-ray examination showed that almost all of these afflicted joints were destroyed. Because of this, for the last eight years she experienced an absolute agony of pain and disability — the last three of them spent in a wheelchair. The doctors considered her chances of recovery — in any way — hopeless. That's because anti-arthritis medications made her sick, and pain killers didn't touch her discomfort. Also, there was so much scarring around her painful joints, there was no place left to cut for more surgery.

Her surgeons had operated on her hands and left them

practically useless. The fingers were so curled up and contracted that she could not pick up a spoon to feed herself. Domestic help, friends, neighbors, and/or relatives came in each day to dress her, get her on the toilet, cook, shop, clean, and help to raise her twin eight-year-old daughters. (Jan's husband died while she was still pregnant.) She was unable to leave the wheelchair for bed unless there was help to bodily lift her tiny frame. She suffered pain all of the time, especially in the knees. Finally, since having that abdominal surgery on January 18, 1989, she had experienced a great deal of embarrassing belching.

Jan Nissen consulted with William J. Faber, D.O. at the Milwaukee Pain Clinic and Metabolic Research Center on March 28, 1989. After examining the patient, evaluating her x-rays, and doing a full history review, Dr. Faber advised her about the many treatment procedures that had to be followed. Eventually a total body reconstructive and neural therapy would have to be carried out along with extensive biological therapy — detoxification and nutritional supplementation — to control the biochemical imbalances brought on by her rheumatoid disease.

Jan listened and said, "I've been through many surgeries, leaving me only worse than before. I'll try your way with injections, Dr. Faber. They certainly can't disable me any more than I already am. I've been through a lot."

Dr. Faber went into his program of restoring Jan Nissen. The injection procedures that he knew would improve her condition followed only after his correction of her biochemical imbalances. He put the patient on a metabolic protocol that proved successful. Then, the osteopath employed injections with lidocaine into her nerves and scars. They were performed to immediately give Jan freedom from indigestion and belching.

After a few weeks on metabolic therapy, some injection sets

of reconstructive therapy were used, and Jan found herself able to bend both of her knees without feeling stabbing pain. Tears of joy rolled down her cheeks as she described her lack of pain to Dr. Faber. Jan realized that she was finally making some headway over the condition instead of growing worse.

She made the 250-mile trip from Wausau, on a regular basis. Each visit to the Milwaukee Pain Clinic found her with a new bit of progress to report. For instance, at the end of the first month her gas and digestive difficulties were gone completely and for good. In another month she could independently move in bed without assistance.

The injection treatment was expanded to her ankles, right knee, wrists, fingers, elbows, and neck. Each time more movement and less pain resulted. Her occipital nerves at the base of her skull were injected around the fourth month, and this gave her such energy that she only took one short nap in a day instead of three longer ones. Her menstrual period, which had discontinued five years before, returned to a normal monthly flow. Her arthritis stopped flaring, and her migraine headaches ceased. Her tinnitus (ringing in the ears) decreased considerably. Injections in the cranial area correct or lessen tinnitis, too.

Just six weeks prior to this writing (November 1, 1989), she received her first reconstructive therapy set of injections into her right hip. She got a "take" and found herself within the week able to pivot on her right leg. She felt more strength than ever before and less pain from rheumatoid arthritis. Jan wanted to try dancing, but her left knee with its artificial prosthesis planted inside didn't permit her the security of standing on two legs.

She admits that the reconstructive injections hurt. However, Jan says, "I'm willing to put up with a few minutes of needle discomfort for a whole lot of joint improvement each time they are over. I can see myself cooking, cleaning, walking, dressing, and just doing everything again the way I used to. I don't feel hopeless anymore. I can't wait to get more treatment because it just keeps me feeling better and better. If it weren't for Dr. Faber and his special injection techniques, I'd be living in a nursing home with pain — totally helpless. But that's not my destiny any more."

An attractive 43-year-old unmarried psychological counselor, Merna Ralston, from Los Angeles, was traveling throughout the United States giving lectures and doing private counseling on mental imagery, Sylva Mind Control, and transcendental meditation. She was a great exponent of the New Age concept of healing and self-improvement. Her very successful occupation came to a sudden end with a serious motor vehicle accident in which she suffered back injuries. After eight weeks of hospitalization, she was unable to walk on her own, and used a wheelchair or walked with the support of a friend. The psychologist had severe low back pain and excruciating neck pain that seemed never to leave her.

The neck discomfort started gradually following her trauma and then increased in severity over the following weeks and continued into the second year until it became intolerable. Ms. Ralston found herself unable to sit for any period of time longer than thirty minutes because of penetrating needle-like sensations in the injured areas. This famous psychologist had to forego her professional counseling with individuals because the usual one- on-one counseling session took a minimum of 55 minutes. She had a 75 percent loss of motor and sensory function in the lower extremities and repeated bouts of vertigo. A few times she actually fell down because the dizziness made her feel as if the ground came up to meet her.

Initially she was seen both by a neurosurgeon and an orthopedic surgeon. A magnetic resonance imaging (MRI) diagnostic procedure had revealed separately to the two specialists that the patient was the victim of double herniated discs in the lumbar spine, and one bulging disc, which exerted some apparent pressure on the cauda equina. The cauda equina is a bundle of nerve roots from the lumbar, sacral, and coccygeal spinal nerves that descend nearly vertically from the spinal cord until they reach their respective openings in the vertebral column. Ms. Ralston's difficulty with walking was diagnosed as bilateral (on both sides) radiculopathy of the sciatic nerve, caused by multilevel lumbar disc herniation.

She learned to walk with a cane, and approximately one-and-one- half-years after the accident her condition appeared to gradually improve. Then, in April 1988, she was flying from Los Angeles to Albuquerque to visit friends in Santa Fe. The airport in Albuquerque was undergoing major construction work. As Ms. Ralston was walking through the airport building, a temporary wall collapsed without warning and buried the patient beneath it. There was apparent injury, but the woman shrugged off assistance and proceeded with her travel plans without accepting immediate medical attention from the airport authorities.

Thereafter, however, her neck pain came back stronger than ever and remained with her constantly. She experienced frequent headaches, too, which settled mostly in the occipital area and appeared to be associated with more vertigo. Furthermore, a new symptom of chronic sporadic confusion arose for Ms. Ralston. When she was driving her car, she had difficulty getting oriented, and more often than not she got lost even in a familiar environment. It was usual for her to require directions from strangers on the street even in neighborhoods she should have known well.

Ms. Ralston visited a well-known neurologist in Los Angeles, who had graduated from Stanford University. He requested that she undergo another MRI of the cervical spine, which revealed a severe disc herniation at the level of the fifth and sixth cervical vertebrae, with pressure on the spinal cord. He recommended that she have immediate neck surgery. But since she was once again experiencing frequent episodes of being unable to walk without help, the neurologist additionally suspected that she had multiple sclerosis. A third MRI of the brain and spinal fluid clearly indicated that she was beset by a severe degree of demyelinating disease. MS was diagnosed as being a complicating factor for her.

Multiple sclerosis (disseminated sclerosis) is a chronic disease of the nervous system affecting young and middle-aged adults. The myelin sheaths surrounding nerves in the brain and spinal cord are damaged, which affects the function of the nerves involved. The course of the illness is characterized by recurrent relapses followed by remissions. The disease affects different parts of the brain and spinal cord, resulting in typically scattered symptoms. These include unsteady gait and shaky movements of the limbs (ataxia), rapid involuntary movements of the eyes (nystagmus), defects in speech pronunciation (dysarthria), spastic weakness, and retrobulbar neuritis. The underlying cause of the nerve damage remains unknown but evidence points to the patient's abnormal response to a viral infection.

Another physician, an internist, suggested observing the progression of her illness. A fourth specialist, a neurologist, considered immunosuppressive therapy for this woman. Merna Ralston refused such a radical, toxic treatment , and attempted to find solace on her own in various alternative methods of healing. In a short time, for instance, she visited two chiropractors, one acupuncturist, and several complementary method healers such as an herbalist and a Christian scientist, but these practitioners brought her temporary or no improvement.

At the end of July, 1989, in her ever-present search for treatment, she consulted the reconstructive therapist Dietrich K. Klinghardt, M.D., Ph.D. board certified diplomate in the pain management specialties of neurological and orthopaedic medicine. Dr. Klinghardt is medical director of the Santa Fe Pain Center in Santa Fe, New Mexico. Ms. Ralston had read an article about Dr. Klinghardt's work in one of the local New Age newspapers. When she arrived at his pain center, the doctor saw that she clearly had a neurological gait, as typical for multiple sclerosis. She could only walk with somebody holding onto her on one side, plus she had to use a cane for support on the other side. However, her most severe complaint was the enormous, unrelenting, severe neck pain, and the nonstop headache, which by now felt as though it was stabbing into every corner of the cranium. Merna Ralston said that she thought her case was hopeless, and death would be welcome as an end to her chronic joint pain.

The neurological signs for which Dr. Klinghardt checked were consistent with a central disc herniation at the fifth and sixth cervical vertebrae, with bilateral weakness of the biceps muscle (in both arms), and loss of the biceps reflex. In the lower extremity, she showed full muscle strength in all of the muscle groups tested. Still, there were scattered areas of insensitivity of the skin to light touch and pin-prick, in a nondermatomal fashion. She also had a positive Babinski sign bilaterally. The Babinski sign indicates that there is disease in the brain or spinal cord (such as MS). It is elicited by drawing a bluntly pointed object along the outer border of the sole of the foot from the heel to the little toe. The normal flexor response is a bunching and downward movement of the toes. An upward movement of the great toe is called an extensor response or Babinski reflex.

She received osteopathic manipulation of the cervical spine, performed under traction, followed by four sets of injections to the spine. Dr. Klinghardt gave her the treatments at weekly intervals. The cervical facet joints, the interspinous ligaments, and the supraspinous ligaments were injected from the level C-1 through T-1 on both sides of the patient's spinal cord. During each treatment, 20 cc of the Ongley solution was used (consisting of the biologic ingredients phenol, glycerin, and dextrose, with lidocaine).

After only three weeks, perhaps even to the surprise of Dr. Klinghardt, Ms. Ralston was completely pain free in the cervical area. Her neck pain had simply disappeared, never to return. Her headaches went away as well, and they have not to this time returned either. In fact, after just the second series of proliferating injections, Dr. Klinghardt reports, the patient was able to walk with merely a cane. Amazingly, since the fourth treatment series, she has not used the cane either and literally threw it away. Her vertigo disappeared, too.

"By mid-August," Dr. Klinghardt tells us in a letter, "I started to address the patient's low back pain. A caudal epidural injection amounting to 30 cc of 0.5 percent Novocaine™ [neural therapy about which the authors are writing a second book] was given. This led to marked increase in sensitivity and feeling on the surface of both lower extremities. [Remember that the woman had lost 75 percent of her feeling in her lower limbs.] This was followed with an adjunctive course of reconstructive therapy injections to the lumbosacral area, also given at weekly intervals.

"After the third injection series, her overall low back pain, which had been there unintermittently for four years was reduced by at least 80 percent. I expect further improvement with maybe two more treatments with reconstructive therapy. I expect that the pain relief that the patient has experienced will be lasting," said Dr. Klinghardt. "I have no explanation why the symptoms that are obviously attributable to the multiple sclerosis have also improved. But the woman should no longer consider that her case is hopeless."

When Magnolia Watts was eight years old, she dashed into the street after a ball and was hit by a car The injury to this little girl's head, neck, shoulders, and back was devastating. Six of her seven cervical vertebrae were fractured, and a cervical fusion was performed in the hospital, where she remained for eight months. In fact, the emergency room staff of the hospital to which she was first taken said that they had no facilities to give sufficient care for such a seriously traumatized patient. In a second hospital little Maggy lingered for six months between life and death until she came out of the crisis. She recuperated for another two months.

For half-a-year more she wore a metal neck brace supporting her head and neck down to her midback. She was unable to walk, and it took her nearly two years to again learn how to ambulate on two feet. She did well until at age 35, in April 1984 while performing her usual occupation as an assembler and welder of parts in a Watertown, Wisconsin small household appliances factory, Mrs. Watts, a woman grown tall and shapely, was once again struck by pain in her left arm, hand, upper back, neck, and head. Her fingers tingled and felt numb alternately. She could no longer perform tasks on the assembly line that required dexterity.

The physician who dispensed industrial medicine to sick or injured employees of the woman's small appliance factory, put her in the hospital where she remained for one week. The misdiagnosis rendered there was "arthritis, that you'll have to live with. There's nothing you can do," Mrs. Watts told us. "I went to a second hospital connected with a medical school and stayed there for another five days. The orthopedic and neurological specialists who checked me over said I didn't just have arthritis but rather I had spinal nerve problems connected with my fused vertebrae. A myelogram proved that she had herniated cervical disc involvement at the base of her cervical fusion. They wanted to give me steel rods in my upper back and a cervical disc surgery. But in explaining what the surgery would do, they got me frightened. Their warnings were that these operations could paralyze me as a result of all the tooling around inside my spine. I didn't want to take that chance.

"I left that hospital and consulted with an another orthopedic surgeon who had a good reputation. He operated on actors, politicians, and sports figures. That doctor looked me over and said that my case was 'intriguing' and a challenging solution was at hand. He wanted to do more surgery on my cervical spine — also to remove the disc and to put metal rods in my neck that would make me a 'stickwoman' — hold me exactly straight as a board so I'd have no more movement. I refused the operation and left that doctor forever," Mrs. Watts said. "But the pains in my back and down my back brought me to tears almost every day, because they were getting worse. I couldn't sleep at night, the hurt was so bad. No amount of pain-killing pills did any good. In fact, I was worried about becoming a junky because I was relying on the many doctors' prescription drugs so much just to get through the day.

"More consultations during the next couple of months gave me the feeling that my case was hopeless. All of the specialists either wanted to shoot me with cortisone, put surgical rods into my back, and remove a cervical disc so that I wouldn't bend left and right or up and down anymore," the woman explained. "I just had to keep looking for help, but I did tell my husband that I didn't believe there was any to be found."

Mrs. Watts traveled next to a famous medical clinic out of state at which the clinic chart diagnosis was "cerebral spinal fluid leak believed to be causing her headaches. Additionally she has C-6, C-7 radiculopathy. " Again she was offered surgical implantation of steel rods and cervical disc surgery as the ultimate means of pain relief. She turned down the procedure once more and simply gave up hope of getting rid of her neck pain and headaches.

"My husband and I saw Dr. Faber being interviewed on a television show coming out of Milwaukee. He was talking about reconstructive therapy, something we had never heard of before, but it sounded like the treatment might do me some good. That was in October, 1984, and I had already been suffering the pains of the damned for eight months. So I picked up the telephone right then and made an appointment for consultation at the Milwaukee Pain Clinic," said Magnolia Watts. "It turns out this was the wisest decision I ever made besides accepting my husband's marriage proposal."

Listening to the woman's medical history and learning of her symptoms, Dr. Faber understood the kind of trouble Mrs. Watts was experiencing. He examined her by palpation, looked at the CAT scan, myelogram, and x-ray films she brought in. He recognized that she had C-7, T-1 disk herniation and cervical vertebrae fusion. The neurological report accompanying her diagnostic films indicated that Mrs. Watts had "hypermobility of C-7 and T-1, complete surgical fusion from C-2 to C-7, intervertebral foramina narrowing from C-1 to C-6, scoliosis of the dorsal spine, and disrupted disks in the lumbar spine at L-4/ L-5 and L-5/S-1. Limited turning of the head with neck pain is the predominant symptom. The patient shows left hemiphoresis from spinal cord disease secondary to trauma. I believe," wrote the consultant, "that the patient's problem is musculoskeletal primary with secondary neurological."

"After Dr. Faber gave me the first set of injections of neural therapy, the pain was gone within a few minutes. I had no more headache. My neck pain went away," continued Mrs.

Watts. "I went back to the clinic a week later, but my pain was still gone. The treatments continued, for they were especially intended to rid me of the finger numbness and tingling. At the spot in my back where the old bony fusion ended I had felt weak, but the proliferating injections made the back and neck feel strong.

"I had been out of work since my fingers acted up in April. Now, nearly nine months later, I could use my hands again. The pins and needles and numbness disappeared. I went back to work without that old hopeless feeling that my case was beyond a solution," she said.

"I had no side effects from the reconstructive therapy; was free of pain; felt stronger in my spine, and could move my limbs with agility. Now, because of my particular neck fusion problem, I take reconstructive therapy periodically to continue strengthening the spine," explained Magnolia Watts. "That's why I'm at the Milwaukee Pain Clinic, today, five years later. Since having the recurrence of my symptoms and their being made to disappear permanently, I don't ever want them to return. I haven't felt any discomfort during all this time, but taking more reconstructive therapy is like an insurance policy that no trouble will strike me again."

A 58-year-old homemaker, Hannah Wisner of Covington, Kentucky, has suffered from osteoarthritis and osteoporosis since 1960. The thinning of her vertebrae caused her to walk in a position so bent over at the neck and midback that she had difficulty seeing where she was going. Mrs. Wisner found difficulty lying on her back because of the curvature of her spine. It was much more than the typical "dowager's hump" that besets many postmenopausal women. Rather, the woman had osteoporosis that disabled her in the extreme. Her orthopedist commented to a colleague one day in her presence that "most people who have the severity of this lady's osteoporotic problem can't even stand on two feet."

Osteoporosis is a condition in which the protein framework (matrix) of the bones become increasingly porous and brittle because of a loss of calcium. This common condition of aging causes bones to fracture more easily. When the spine is involved, the vertebrae collapse, causing curvature and backache as well as decrease in stature. In women so affected, osteoporosis is associated with the postmenopausal decrease in estrogen.

A chiropractor who adjusted her twice weekly enabled the patient to continue to function in a limited way. His manipulations gave Mrs. Wisner temporary relief from the pain that passed in waves along the course of her spine. The relief lasted about one day. At home she could not make her bed in the morning or get out of the bathtub without help. One of the most heart-wrenching problems for her was that Mrs. Wisner could not hug her grandchildren, because the pressure of their arms around her body hurt so badly.

During the previous twenty-eight years of suffering with her condition, Mrs. Wisner had gone through a host of doctors looking for that one medical specialist who would find relief for her pain and body distortion. Hopelessness fell upon her when it finally became apparent that usual medical practices held no such relief. Steadily worsening disability and increasing pain was in store for her, Mrs. Wisner knew. That's the reason it took several months of urging by her daughter before this woman decided that she would try just one more therapeutic approach to solving her problem.

The daughter, Mrs. Connie Ciaglia, the wife of a plumber, had settled in Mt. Cory, Ohio right after she graduated from Bluffton College. Her alma mater is located in Bluffton, Ohio, the town in which family practice specialist L. Terry Chappell, M.D. practices reconstructive therapy. Dr. Chappell is medical director of the Celebration of Health Center. Mrs. Ciaglia had

274

heard an enormous number of excellent reports from friends and neighbors pertaining to musculoskeletal recoveries being achieved by Dr. Chappell. No other physician in the area seemed to be employing reconstructive therapy. The daughter persuaded Mrs. Wisner to take the three-hour drive up Interstate Highway 75 from Covington to Bluffton to receive the doctor's treatment.

Dr. Chappell did an initial thermography study of Mrs. Wisner. As we described earlier, thermography measures an apparently objective parameter — change in tissue perfusion — that may be associated with pain, but does not measure the degree of pain. It is recommended for use when the doctor suspects deafferentation pain (a loss of the sensory nerve fibers from a portion of the body) such as in reflex sympathetic dystrophy, causalgia, or nerve root irritation. In their early stages none of these conditions show x-ray, electromylographic, or nerve conduction velocity changes.

Thermography is excellent for chronic joint pain diagnosis because it detects changes in blood flow in the top layer of the skin. It uses an infrared camera to measure body surface temperatures, thus indirectly allowing assessment of sympathetic nerve function. The affected area will be at least 1 degree C (1.8 degrees F) cooler or warmer than the opposite, anatomically identical area. The technique is non-invasive, rarely involves skin-to-instrument contact, and is not particularly time- consuming or expensive. It can be repeated as often as necessary and causes no discomfort or danger to the patient.

Some studies have shown that thermographs can detect otherwise overlooked organic disorders, particularly reflex sympathetic dysfunction that may easily be misdiagnosed as psychogenic pain (where the doctor thinks, "It's all in your head).[1]

The thermographic study conducted by Dr. Chappell of

Mrs. Wisner was interpreted at the thermographic laboratories of Thermascan, Incorporated, located in the Detroit metropolitan area. Laboratory director Philip Hoekstra, III, Ph.D., on August 2, 1989, submitted his report to Dr. Chappell. Dr. Hoekstra confirmed the following:

> Hyperthermia, which is indicative of severe inflammation, was evident in both sides of the patient's neck, extending into the upper back. There were also irritated areas alongside the vertebral bones at the fourth and fifth cervical vertebrae as well as the fourth and fifth lumbar vertebrae in the midback. The right facet or lateral joint of the fifth lumbar and first sacral vertebrae were prominently inflamed. The mechanism of pathology was thought to be osteoarthritis and osteoporosis, as previously mentioned, and it was assumed to have been aggravated by a motor vehicle accident that she had been subjected to in 1987.

Because he believed that she would respond quite well to the treatment, Dr. Chappell administered reconstructive therapy to Mrs. Wisner. After the first five visits that she made to the Celebration of Health Center for a series of proliferating injections, the patient noticed a dramatic improvement in her ability to function.

She declared that her neck could turn more freely. She could bend and touch her toes, whereas before the woman could reach down only two feet from the floor. While her back was bent, she explained, it had stiffened in that position and was inflexibly rigid — but not any more. Additionally, Mrs. Wisner found herself doing personal tasks that had been physically impossible before. Now she could readily make her bed after arising. She could also get out of the bathtub without any difficulty.

Astonishing her husband, she even tried riding a bicycle and managed it very well. "I hadn't thought about bicycle-riding since I was a young girl," said Hannah Wisner, "but now with the reconstructive therapy, such an endeavor seemed to be like the ultimate test. I did it and, with that first-time bicycling, which I do now several times a week, my hopelessness disappeared."

Her chiropractor continued to adjust her back and was amazed as well at how well his adjustments were now holding. Pain never was a factor for her anymore. She went for his adjustments merely because they made her feel good and lifted her spirits. On her own she could climb onto his treatment table without difficulty.

Just prior to her fifth visit for reconstructive therapy, Mrs. Wisner slipped on a walnut in her kitchen and fell to the floor, bumping into her doorway frame. Surprising everyone, she felt no stiffness or pain after this trauma. Pain in the area that had been inflamed previously, did not reappear. Her spine had developed a flexibility that allowed her to rebound from the incident.

In October, 1989 Dr. Chappell called for the patient to have a repeat thermography test. This showed much reduction of inflammation from the prior study. Her osteoarthritis has dissipated, and the osteoporotic bones seem to be firming up of their own accord at their ligamentous attachments. Stronger ligaments seem to be adding to the strength of her backbones.

The technical aspects of this case aside, however, most precious to Hannah Wisner is that her grandchildren can now hug her as hard as they want. She feels no pain whatsoever — only joy.

Why "Hopeless" Cases Don't Remain Hopeless Anymore

Why does reconstructive therapy take hopelessness and turn it into joy? Why is reconstructive therapy truly the most magnificent ligament, tendon, and joint treatment ever to be developed from the minds of the masters in medicine? The main reason is that each application of proliferating solution naturally produces more structure in the connective tissues.

Employing the injection technique is like hiring a mason to build a garden wall. The longer he works the more layers of bricks are going to be laid down. Without connective tissue structure, the body would fall apart. It's all held together by this connective tissue that supports, binds, or separates more specialized tissues and organs, or functions as packing tissue for the body. It consists of an amorphous ground substance of mucopolysaccharides in which may be embedded white (collagenous), yellow (elastic), and reticular fibers, fat cells, fibroblasts, mast cells, and macrophages. Variations in chemical composition of the ground substance and in the proportions and quantities of cells and fibers give rise to tissues of widely differing characteristics, including bone, cartilage, tendons, and ligaments as well as adipose, areolar, and elastic tissues.

In connective tissue, the cells are separated by relatively large amounts of material outside the cell walls. The proliferants, upon injection, become part of this external fluid material that surrounds the cells. It enters them by osmosis through the cellular membranes and stimulates fibroblastic growth. Collagen, for instance, the white fibers of albuminlike connective tissue in cartilage and the organic substance of bones, it's conjectured, may be converted into gelatin by the proliferant so as to make it more amenable to inflammation-reduction.

Making the structure of connective tissue stronger by injectable proliferation, causes it to perform its job of supporting the bones of joints better. It is because of structure that the body resists the constant forces of gravity. Gravity pulls at us with tremendous force which we must fight constantly. Its forces, if not resisted by structure, cause a widening and compression (see Figure 41). With joint impairment, reconstructive

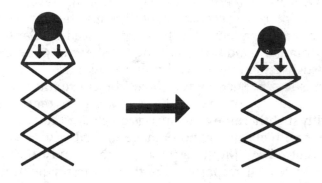

Response to Gravity Causes Structures to Become Shorter and Wider

Figure 41

279

therapy comes to the rescue, because it is anti-gravity treatment literally holding up the body.

Reconstructive therapy acts like a perfect splint. You don't have to strap it on and have it pinch, pull, push, slip, stick, or bite you as do so many braces, supports, and paddings. Reconstructive therapy turns out to be the correct size as a supportive measure — extra strong. Remember that experiments on laboratory animals have provided us with proof that reconstructive therapy increases ligamentous strength by 40 percent over normal. It's permanent strengthening, too.

Dr. William J. Faber reports that now, in his seventh year of practicing intensive reconstructive therapy, he has never witnessed a single patient who has experienced a relapse to his or her original condition once he or she has gone through reconstructive therapy to maximum rebuilding.

Reconstructive therapy reinforces the entire interconnective articular network of the joint structure. It accomplishes this task with such harmony and precision that wonderful successes result with absolutely no damage to the body.

Dr. Wilfred W. Mittlestadt whose case study opened this chapter, states, "If reconstructive therapy has side effects that are harmful, I certainly would be aware of them. I've received thousands of individual needlings with hundreds of proliferants — intensive injections throughout my damaged spine — with never any ill effect. And I'm 83 years old. Time has shown me, after over 50 years of practicing medicine, that the more medications and surgery you take the worse the complications — not so with reconstructive therapy. As long as the body has biochemical healing abilities it just produces stronger structure and permanent ligamentous benefits by receiving reconstructive therapy."

Chapter Sixteen

Therapeutic Myths of Cortisone and Exercise

Before the advent of reconstructive therapy, no one in medicine really knew how to spell relief for chronic joint pain. Even now, in fact, various pain clinics don't even use the same definitions in describing the pain that penetrates joints and creates agony for myriad numbers of people who are unresponsive to conventional modes of treatment.

The highly competitive pain-killer market shows what advertising dollars can buy. In the spring of 1987 the pharmaceutical industry's trade newspaper reported that the five leading product lines (Tylenol™, Anacin™, Bayer Aspirin™, Bufferin™, and Excedrin™) spent approximately $750 million in advertising during 1986. With their massive effort, these few products alone captured nearly $4 billion in sales, or two-thirds of all that American medical consumers spent on over-the-counter (OTC) and prescription drugs to relieve pain. Most of this pain is directly related to chronic joint subluxations from ligaments that are lax, weakened, or torn.

According to the August 28, 1989 issue of *Medical World News*, an estimated 80 million Americans, many on a tireless quest for help, visit over 1,000 pain clinics.[1] They engage in the conventional treatments of drugs, bed rest, physical therapy, orthopedic surgery, neurological surgery, traction, psychotropics, and group therapy. Or, they will possibly pursue the less traditional forms of pain therapy such as acupuncture, acupressure, shiatsu, reflexology adjustments, myotherapy, Rolfing, the Feldenkrais technique, polarity therapy, orgone therapy, the Alexander technique, the Mensendieck System, the Lotte Berk Method, chiropractic, Swedish massage, biofeedback, Bioenergetics, hypnosis, Christian Science prayer, or some other pain-alleviating procedure.

The unfortunate patients with pain habitually take anti- inflammatory drugs such as aspirin, cortisone, Motrin™, Nuprin™, Nalfon™, Clinoril™, Feldene™, Naprosyn™, Indocin™, Tolectin™, or the equivalent in huge quantities. They may be addicted to narcotics and tranquilizers, such as the woman described in a clinical journal report by Johns Hopkins University hospital. She sought treatment at the pain clinic there, and her case history revealed that the poor soul had taken 28,000 pain pills in 1988 alone. Or, there was another woman who entered the University of Washington clinic after having undergone 44 major surgeries on her back.

Joint pain is the most common disability in the world. Sufferers of chronic pain spent over $70 billion for professional medical or complementary health care assistance in 1989. To exploit this market for pain relief, American anesthesiologists have added new requirements to their specialty board — pain management training and testing.

A pain-sufferer can buy treatment almost anywhere in surroundings ranging from a one-person acupuncture office upstairs from a restaurant in Chinatown to a chrome, plastic and steel university-affiliated comprehensive pain center staffed with 100 fulltime professionals, some of them medical school professors. There also are syndrome-oriented facilities — back clinics, headache clinics — and the offices of private physicians who have chosen to specialize in managing all types of pain. The facilities for pain relief are variable, some colorful, others sterile, and all of them interesting.

"A good half of them I wouldn't send my pet to," said

Steven Brena, M.D. Dr. Brena, chairman of the Pain Control and Rehabilitation Institute of Georgia in Decatur, claims that at least 15 Georgia facilities billing themselves as pain clinics are "fronts" for physicians to perform nerve blocks, acupuncture, or surgery. Even university affiliation does not guarantee good pain care, he added.

The Cortisone Ripoff

With all the potential for patient exploitation or therapeutic mismanagement in cases of musculoskeletal or myofascial pain syndromes due to trauma, the biggest ripoff is injectable or orally-administered cortisone. Yes, of the many drugs given for the relief of chronic joint pain, the one most harmfully employed by many health professionals is cortisone, its derivatives, and its associated compounds. This is not an OTC drug but rather one that is studiously prescribed by uninformed or misinformed physicians.

Corticosteroid products that are supposed to relieve pain by their anti-inflammatory effect actually bring into being new damage to the joint's ligamentous attachments. The corticosteroid drugs cause dissolution of ligament and tendon attachments — an actual liquifaction of the fibrous tissues at and around bony articulations. The 1989, 49th Edition of the *Physician's Desk Reference* clearly states, "Frequent intra-articular injection [with cortisone] may result in damage to joint tissues."

Furthermore, corticosteroids cause osteoporosis or softening of bones, making them weak and more easily fractured. Injection of a steroid into any infected site is bad medical practice and outright dangerous. Cortisone can spread the infection. Also a marked increase in pain accompanied by local swelling, further restriction of joint motion, fever, and malaise are suggestive of septic arthritis spread by the cortisone.

The side effects of corticosteroids are numerous, yet many

physicians are in the habit of employing them. The doctors are inadvertently engaging in the cortisone ripoff because they seem unaware of the lack of evidence of the drug's effectiveness and that it definitely causes harm to the recipients' joints. Still, these physicians continue to inject the potent remedy or prescribe oral administration because of old information that lingers from the years when cortisone was a so-called "miracle drug."

Another reason that doctors still erroneously use this drug for chronic joint pain is that cortisone preparations remain under the United States and international patent protection. Pharmaceutical companies aggressively market corticosteroids to physicians. Very considerable profit is built into the pricing of patented corticosteroids.

Many physicians think that if they judge a drug to work, even if scientific studies show it does not — such as the research being done at the University of Wisconsin Medical School on the deleterious effects of cortisone when used for the treatment of chronic joint pain — they have the right to prescribe the drug. A graphic example can be given of this wrong-headed thinking. Early in the 1950s, diethylstilbesterol (DES), a corticosteroid, was shown in published, well-controlled studies not to protect women from miscarriage. Nevertheless, even after this time, it was still prescribed to prevent miscarriages in millions of women because some doctors "believed" the drug worked. Each had seen a woman with a miscarriage in a previous pregnancy take DES and avoid a miscarriage during a subsequent pregnancy.

Blinded to the notion that it was not DES, but just the natural variation from one pregnancy to the next, doctors rejected scientific studies in deference to their own personal experience and therefore exposed millions of mothers and children to DES, the effects of which have included cancer, birth defects, and problems with pregnancies. In the same way, this has been proven the case with cortisone for the treatment of chronic joint pain. As in the clinical studies and case histories cited in the following sections, cortisone given for the treatment of tendon, ligament, or joint impairment is often ineffective and even may be destructive.

Published Studies Proving Cortisone Destruction

Writing in the *Archives of Neurology*, D.A. Nelson, M.D. advises his medical colleagues that clinical trials first began in 1960 with methylprednisolone acetate, a corticosteroid known commercially as Depo-Medrol™ administered intrathecally (within the sheath), in an attempt to treat both disc disease and multiple sclerosis. After a few reports of positive results, there began an outpouring of contradictory data, which continues to the present.

During this 28-year time span, researchers who cautiously tested the different theses of improvement began to publish serious warnings of many cortisone complications. For ten years prior to the intraspinal use of methylprednisolone acetate, basic scientists in anesthesiology and neurochemistry had published the following facts:

(1) Methylprednisolone acetate's content of polyethylene glycol raises the risks of using it near the central nervous system.

(2) Deleterious effects follow the use of glycols when they are placed into or near the neuraxis (spinal cord).

(3) Methylpredinisolone acetate contains approximately 30 milligrams (mg) of polyethylene glycol per milliliter (ml).

(4) When that glycol, which is both alcohol and detergent, is injected intraspinally, sterile meningitis, arachnoiditis, or pachymeningitis will occur. It has also been recognized since the 1960s that the epidural space is not wholly separate from the subdural and/or subarachnoid space. Many thousands of arachnoid villi subtend all the membranes from the intrathecal

285

space, and many of these end in the large epidural veins. Therefore, the various spaces and membranes are not only contiguous, but continuous. It follows that an injection of methylprednisolone acetate into the epidural space does not guarantee that it will remain isolated there. Finally, the inadvertency of injections by the epidural route occurs with the following frequency: 40 percent of injections can be inadvertently made into interspinous ligaments (causing the ligaments to dissolve), and 2.5 percent into the subarachnoid space (causing paralysis or death).[2]

Next, a case of Achilles tendon rupture in both legs that simulated peripheral neuropathy was reported by Drs. W. Dickey and V. Patterson, in June 1987. It was a complication of corticosteroid therapy.[3] The effect of Kenalog™, a triamcinolone acetonide cortisone product, administered into the joints or tendons of rat extremities had an effect on the animals' vital organs. These intra-articular injections of the knee joints affected the animals' adrenal glands, liver, and stomach.[4]

Fourth, in a Chinese journal published in April 1987, another case study in a middle-aged man was reported on ruptured achilles tendons from the joint injection of triamcinolone.[5]

Then there was the spontaneous and iatrogenic (doctor-caused) subcutaneous rupture of the tendons of the hand in people and guinea pigs from the injection of methylprednisolone.[6]

Sixth, the ligamentum patella ruptured following local steroid injection in an Australian Rules football player. The relationship between local corticosteroid injection and the rupture of large ligaments and tendons is now well-established. The medical author, Dr. M. Alexeeff, warned in this September 1986 article that careful consideration prior to cortisone injection is strongly suggested because of the risk of rupture of these ligamentous and joint structures.[7]

Three medical authors reported on bilateral simultaneous Achilles tendon rupture in a 44-year-old woman after giving her oral cortisone for the treatment of rheumatoid arthritis. The researchers, who are clinicians, caution that affected persons usually are on chronic steroid treatment and in the fifth to seventh decades of life. The patient may have concomitant systemic disease, and the injury occurs with relatively mild trauma. The goals of treatment are mainly preventative, that is, cessation of steroids as soon as possible and protective bracing of the remaining intact Achilles tendon.[8]

In another 1987 case, after infiltration with cortisone, the adult patient sustained a rupture of the patellar ligament. The steroid employed was betamethasone.[9]

Finally, in the same issue of the journal, the Achilles tendon is reported to have avulsed (ruptured) from a single injection of cortisone in a Danish woman.[10]

Cortisone Pathology Created within Tendons and Cartilage

The harmful side effects of steroids introduced into joints on a repetitive basis is noted by several investigators, including five others indicated in older references.[11, 12, 13, 14, 15] In fact, many medical researchers have reported spontaneous tendon rupture in conjunction with local corticosteroid therapy. These investigators have produced convincing evidence to support the reality that glucocorticoids adversely affect tendons and ligaments, as well.[16, 17, 18, 19, 20, 21]

So, what happens? J.C. Kennedy, M.D., Professor and Chief of the Division of Orthopaedic Surgery, Faculty of Medicine, University of Western Ontario, London, Ontario and R. Baxter Willis, M.D. of the same faculty, presented their conclusions about the villainous effects of cortisone. They said:

- Physiologic doses of local steroid, placed directly into a normal tendon, weaken it significantly for up to four-

287

teen days following the injection.

- The biomechanical disruption is directly related to collagen necrosis.
- Restoration of function, by fourteen days, is due to the formation of relatively acellular, amorphous material, — a precursor of collagen.
- Avoidance of vigorous muscular activity for at least two weeks should be emphasized to the patient receiving local steroids.
- Repetitive injections of local corticosteroids should be avoided.[22]

Case Histories of Damage Done by Steroid Injections on Connective Tissue

Louis J. Unverferth, Clinical Instructor, Division of Orthopedics, The Ohio State University, Columbus, and Melvin L. Olix, Clinical Instructor, Division of Orthopedics and Team Physician at the same institution, presented a series of case histories of damage done by steroid injections on connective tissue of college athletes.[23] For example, a twenty-one-year-old college football player, (place-kicking specialist) developed a painful tenosynovitis of his right Achilles tendon (kicking side) in the fall of 1970. Over a period of nine weeks, the patient received four injections of steroid in and about his painful Achilles tendon. The injections were given approximately two weeks apart. Four weeks after the last injection, following a brief period of improvement, the patient, while attempting to kick off, experienced a sudden onset of severe pain in the right Achilles tendon. The diagnosis of complete rupture of the Achilles tendon was made by Drs. Unverferth and Olix and confirmed at surgery. The tendon was ruptured approximately one inch above its insertion into the heel bone and was markedly frayed. Much hemorrhage was noted. Deposits of yellow substance made up of steroid were found on and within the thickened tendon sheath.

The second case was of a twenty-seven year-old professional basketball player who developed a painful right Achilles tendon in September 1971. He was treated with local injections of steroid on four different occasions. Between the injections of local steroid, the patient was allowed to move around on crutches. Ice packs were applied daily to the right heel. This treatment was discontinued after ten days at which time the athlete attempted to return to competition. After two days of practice, he suffered the same symptoms and the entire treatment was repeated. Two weeks after the fourth local injection of cortisone, while attempting a rebound at the basket, the patient had sudden severe pain in his right calf and heel. The diagnosis of complete rupture of the Achilles tendon was made.

At the time of surgery, the tendon was found to be completely ruptured two inches above its insertion into the heel bone. There was a great deal of tendon sheath thickening and bleeding. Small yellow deposits of cortisone were noted on the subcutaneous tissue and on the tendon sheath.

Three more athletes had these same experiences, a male skier, a young football-playing woman, and a sixty-two-year-old male physician and active tennis player who received twelve local steroid injections for tennis elbow. All of them suffered cortisone damage. Observing these deleterious effects, Drs. Unverferth and Olix decided to do some experimenting on rabbits using local cortisone injections. Here are their findings:

- In the rabbits studied, gastrocnemius [calf muscle] tendons when injected with steroid were shown to have statistically lower moduli of elastic stiffness than tendons injected with saline [salt solution]. Since the moduli of elastic stiffness are valid indicators of ultimate tensile strength, steroid-injected tendons will rupture at lower loads than saline injected tendons.

- Macroscopic as well as microscopic examinations of the steroid- injected tendon indicated that tendon destruction takes place particularly around the pools of deposited steroid.
- The use of local steroid injections in the treatment of tenosynovitis should be abandoned, not only because the steroid injections mask the symptoms of tenosynovitis, giving the patient a false sense of security, but also because local injection of steroid in and about tendon decreases the tensile strength of the tendon and predisposes it to complete rupture.

The Myth of Exercise for Chronic Joint Pain

Down through the ages the body of man has changed. The renowned anthropologist, Estabrooks, speaks of modern man as a mechanical misfit. Over the past ten or fifteen million years the humanoid skeleton has altered a great deal. All animals were originally four-legged beasts. Some, like monkeys, began hopping around on their hind legs. Today man is the only animal that walks and keeps his body erect. Early men always walked with a decided stoop and, when not stooping, leaned forward on a club or a cane.

Such alteration in the posture of the humanoid animal made it necessary for certain portions of the body to change, and some of our joint troubles arise from that fact. Consider joints of the backbone, the value of which lie in their flexibility. If the backbone is absolutely rigid, it is impossible for a person to bend, move, or see well. Therefore, nature never provided for the development of mankind with a rigid spine. Instead, his spine is a spring, somewhat curved like the letter S. The top bulge of the letter S forms the round shoulders that occur in many human beings. The bottom of the letter S is the hollow of the back.

As a human gets older, this spring — the discs in his joints — breaks down, just as do metal springs. Ligaments that hold each of the articulating bones together but separated become too loose and overly relaxed to the point where they do not support the joint. If this laxness happens in the spinal joints, the shoulders become stooped. The hollow of the back first straightens out and, as Estabrooks says, "then hollows the wrong way." In other words, as the peculiar structure of the human spine changes with age, it comes to resemble more and more that of an animal that walks on four feet instead of two. It forms an arch instead of a spring.

When we are young, it is possible for the joints to be self-regulating mechanisms. No spring made by man will last for the human lifetime. In fact, automobile springs, which are subjected to much less strain than an individual's discs, often break down in less than three years.

Chronic joint pain with the resulting "stiffness" of "arthritis" is one of the most frequent complaints of people past their youth. Among the most common remedies suggested for this arthritic stiffness is exercise. The efficacy of exercise is a myth when applied for chronic joint, tendon, and ligament problems. In the short term, so-called therapeutic exercise only serves to increase the pathology producing joint dysfunction. In the long term, exercise will cause greater stiffness by the splinting of joints with metastatic bone deposition improperly laid down. Stimulated osteoblasts (bone-forming cells) are attempting to do the job of worn-out ligaments.

No muscle fibers exist in tendons, ligaments, joints, cartilage, and disks. Exercise is known to stimulate muscle fibers to grow longer because muscles have good blood supplies. Lacking the elasticity of muscle fibers, ligaments, tendons, cartilage, and discs are aggravated and overly stretched. Exercise just makes them weaker. There is no therapeutic effect for joint spacers in vigorous activity and movement, the spacers

291

are only damaged. They heal poorly and fail to respond to exercise because the ligaments, tendons, cartilage, and disks are poorly nourished with blood flow. An axiom in osteopathic medicine is "The rule of the artery is supreme," meaning that good blood flow equals good healing. Reconstructive therapy, by stimulating the inflammation of local tissue repair, gives these body parts poorly supplied with blood a second chance at healing by causing the dilation of blood vessels as well as reconstruction of tissue.

Chronic joint pain is frequently a reflection of stress or strain on particular joints. If there has been any extraordinary pulling or tearing of tendons or ligaments, for instance, by the sudden twisting that occurs in swinging a golf club or the microtrauma connected with repetitive motions performed in the course of wielding a wrench on the assembly line, simple rest of the affected portion until healing occurs may be all the treatment necessary. If the pain is intense and the joint dysfunction more serious, reconstructive therapy is the correct procedure to follow.

Within the last three decades physicians have discovered that the cartilages that act as cushions between articulating bones may be pushed out of place or damaged, resulting in pain on the slightest motion. Reconstructive therapy helps to heal this problem as well.

Using exercise as a therapeutic modality for an impaired joint is a myth that does the patient an injustice. Therapeutic exercise may be useful for remedying the bundles of fibers acting as power units for muscles, but it does nothing to assist in the mending of joints and their ligaments. Exercise acts against ligaments. Chronic joint pain comes from ligaments not doing their assigned jobs, and exercise just goes on to weaken them more. Only avascular (bloodless) fibrous tissue is present in ligaments and tendons, and nothing is there to get larger by exercise.

When the hinge joints of your car door squeak and close only with much resistance, do you open and shut it purposely to make it stronger? No!

Mikhail Baryshnikov, defected to the West in June 1975 while appearing as a guest artist with the Bolshoi Ballet in Toronto. Widely regarded as the Soviet Union's finest male classical stylist, Baryshnikov was quickly engaged for guest appearances by the American Ballet Theater, making his debut on July 27th that same year in New York as Albrecht in *Giselle*, opposite Natalia Makarova, who had defected from the same company four years earlier. Since then Baryshnikov has gone on to tremendous acclaim in the United States making a fortune in films, on the stage, in television, as a dance director, choreographer, and more. In all of this activity his dancing has tuned his body to the height of fitness. Yet, Baryshnikov has undergone four operations on his knees. Common sense alone indicates that exercise has not done anything to strengthen his knee joints or prevented further injury.

Regular ballet exercises give ballerinas agonizingly painful foot troubles of the joints. With all of the exercise tennis players engage in, they should have no difficulties with their elbow or ankle joints. We know that is not true.

Empirical reasoning wins out over the myth of exercise as appropriate treatment for joint disability. It does not work, except for swimming. In swimming, water surrounds the joints and supports them like bracing. It also neutralizes the gravitational effect (see Figure 40 in Chapter 14) which pulls us into shorter heights.

Exercise Is Useful in Conjunction with Proliferating Injections

The only usefulness of exercise in chronic joint pain as applied by a physical therapist is to increase local blood circulation, to preserve mobility, to stretch tight, contracted muscles, and to increase an individual's physical well-being. Strengthening a joint — any joint — does not happen as a result of exercising that joint. So, don't be carried away by the importance of exercise in rehabilitation of your impaired or disabled joints.

Kent Pomeroy, M.D. of Scottsdale, Arizona, in discussions with colleagues at a roundtable of the American Association of Orthopaedic Medicine told of starting patients on an exercise program during or after the use of proliferating injections. Dr. Pomeroy explained:

> I begin my patients on therapeutic exercise immediately when my injection procedure starts. Most of the injection cases that I have treated require some kind of manipulation, some form of additional correction, and the exercises that I give these people are designed to return their position, such as sacroiliac self- rotation. I may wait, however, until the patient is under fairly good pain control, and after four weeks from the most recent injections, before I let them return to heavy athletic activities, or heavy work activities. Unless, of course, they are professional athletes and this is something that they can't wait very long to get back into. Then you just have to work with that.

Chapter Seventeen

Reconstructive Therapy as Complementary Medicine

Around the world medical care takes many forms including homeopathic medicine, naturopathic medicine, chiropractic, allopathic medicine, osteopathic medicine, Chinese herbal medicine, acupuncture, and at least a dozen others. In the United States, anything other than allopathic medicine is considered to be on the fringe of appropriate practice. Allopathy is this country's establishment medicine that comes out of academic study, utilizing the scientific method — the dominant or conventional way of dispensing health care. This so-called orthodox medicine is accepted in hospitals, taught in medical schools, approved by the American Medical Association, paid for by third-party health insurance carriers, legitimized by the U.S. Government, and subsidized by the pharmaceutical industry.

Still, there are two other types or philosophies of modern medicine made available to the public by conventionally-trained physicians. Called (1) alternative medicine and (2) complementary medicine, they are just as important to the health and welfare of the medical consumer.

The first one, alternative medicine, is mutually exclusive from orthodox practices that ordinarily are employed in American allopathic medicine. It is an alternative to conventional methods, not accepted by the establishment and seldom if ever taught as part of the medical school curriculum. The alternative techniques of healing come from several sources, as for instance new age concepts, proven usage from the East, old wives tales that work, and researched notions of individual physicians who have made clinical observations and repeat a particular therapeutic program because it has produced beneficial effects for other patients besides those being given current attention.

Complementary medicine uses more biological components than allopathy and is the synthesis of both medical orthodoxy and alternatives. For example, a traditionally-practicing physician who boldly incorporates a medical alternative such as suggesting his patient take quantities of garlic daily instead of his prescribing an anti-hypertensive drug for lowering high blood pressure is practicing complementary medicine. In contrast, a homeopathic medical doctor (H.M.D.) — considered an alternativist by allopaths — who seeks immediate alleviation of pain for his patient's headache and suggests the taking of aspirin, also is practicing complementary medicine.

A physician — either a traditional or nontraditional practitioner — who applies reconstructive therapy is practicing complementary medicine. As a complementary treatment method, reconstructive therapy is a compromise answer to the question, should the physician focus on the patient or the patient's disease? Reconstructive therapy responds well to this debate that has raged from the beginnings of medical history when the Hippocratic philosophy centered on the patient and the rival Cnidian philosophy focused on the disease. Perhaps once considered experimental or an "alternative," reconstructive therapy is now part of the newly emerging biological or complementary medicine.

Reconstructive Therapy Adapted by Osteopathic Medicine

Reconstructive therapy fits well into the osteopathic medical philosophy which stresses the unity of all body systems.

Osteopathic physicians also emphasize the musculoskeletal system, "holistic medicine," plus proper nutrition and environmental factors. They bring a "hands-on" approach to medical practice and view manipulation or palpation as an aid to the diagnosis and treatment of various illnesses.

Reconstructive therapy is a holistic and biological way of treating chronic impairments of tendons, ligaments, and joints. Holistic medicine is almost synonymous with the term alternative medicine , and it further means treating the whole person and/or considering each individual as a whole but separate entity as was taught by Hippocrates around 400 B.C. Holism is an opposing concept to allopathic specialization and oftentimes is fallaciously denigrated as "quackery" by health care practitioners active in medical politics. Ironically, establishment medicine is adapting the holistic concept as its own by reintroducing the medical specialty of family practice to replace the old time horse-and-buggy doctors of decades gone by.

Today, the one branch of mainstream medicine that follows the Hippocratic approach most closely is osteopathic medicine. Currently, some 27,500 American osteopathic physicians and surgeons practice holistic medicine by offering the public a different dimension in medical care as compared to the drug-oriented (M.D.) methods of allopathic medicine.

Doctors of Osteopathic Medicine (D.O.s) are fully licensed and recognized physicians whose manner of diagnosis and treatment was founded on the Missouri frontier in 1874. Dr. Andrew Taylor Still was an individualistic and strong-willed M.D. who was rightly dissatisfied with the ineffectiveness of 19th Century medicine. He decried the rudimentary drugs and surgery of the day and saw many people, including his own three children, die from serious diseases. Concepts such as anesthesia, sterile surgery, antiseptics, antibiotics, correct nutrition, injection therapy, and x-rays were not imagined in the 1870s.

In response, Dr. Still founded a philosophy of medicine that harkened back to Hippocrates, with its central emphasis on the unity of the body. He identified the musculoskeletal system as a key element of health, a principal that is gaining acceptance with M.D.s now. He recognized the body's capability to heal itself. He stressed preventive medicine, eating properly, and keeping fit, which mainstream America wholeheartedly embraced in the 1970s.

Dr. Still identified palpation and the human touch as vital to gaining patient confidence and providing effective medical care. He stressed manipulation as a less-intrusive form of diagnosis and treatment. Currently, many people seek procedures and therapies that are less-invasive and less likely to escalate cost or cause side effects. D.O.s, with their M.D. counterparts, offer mainstream medical care — but with a difference.

Paul H. Goodley, M.D. of Phoenix, Arizona, past president of the American Association of Orthopaedic Medicine, in his 1984 post inaugural address to that august body, said: "Palpatory skill is the quintessence, the pure distillation, the most vital ingredient, the primal identifier, the fundamental of orthopaedic medicine. And I submit that its presence, or its absence, is potent and sufficient to influence physicians and their attitudes in their subsequent acts."

Reconstructive Therapy Fits Well into Osteopathy

Osteopathy emphasizes that all body systems, including the musculoskeletal system, operate in unison — and disturbances in one system can alter the functions of other systems. By recognizing the close relationship between body structure and organic functioning, the D.O. has a broader base for treating the whole patient. The osteopathic doctor not only acknowledges the interdependence of all parts of the complex machine — the human body — but also considers the patient's mental and emotional status. In addition, he or she pays attention to the relationship of the patient to his or her home environment, job, and other factors that affect health.

Reconstructive therapy fits well into the osteopathic concept, since the musculoskeletal system is central to the patient's well-being. This system includes the bones, muscles, tendons, connective tissues, ligaments, nerves, and spinal column — over 60 percent of the body mass. The musculoskeletal framework is far more than an anatomical rack on which the other organs are hung. It works in concert with all other organs. It responds every time a breath is drawn or any other body movement occurs. Besides being prone to mechanical disorders, the musculoskeletal system reflects many internal illnesses and may aggravate or accelerate the process of disease in the circulatory, lymphatic, nervous, and other body systems.

Another osteopathic concept is that the body has a natural tendency toward health, as well as the capacity to resist disease and to heal itself. The body's own healing power, *vis medicatrix naturae*, is a main principle of osteopathic medicine and a basic condition of all diagnosis and treatment. Therefore, osteopathic practice is designed to support, stimulate, and initiate the body's tendency toward health.

Reconstructive therapy fits these osteopathic concepts inasmuch as in addition to treating specific health problems, the professional goal is to help every patient function at his or her highest level of efficiency. There is a fundamental concern with preventive medicine, proper nutrition, and keeping the patient well. The reconstructive therapist applies all of those programs for high-level wellness. He also engages in sports medicine as a natural outgrowth of osteopathic practice, which focuses on the musculoskeletal system, injection therapy, manipulation, diet, exercise, and fitness. Many professional sports team physicians, Olympic physicians, and personal sports medicine doctors are D.O.s who make use of all types of complementary medicine, including reconstructive therapy.

Importance of Reconstructive Therapy for Work-Related Injuries

This book would be incomplete without information about the therapy's use for work-related injuries, especially those traumas that take place on the job among blue-collar workers. The blue collar worker, and even the white collar worker, who gets hurt on the job or through accidental injury, frequently receives a raw deal from social services, in particular from Worker's Compensation Insurance coverage. The physically injured party faces difficulty in regaining health and happiness because of the system of compensation. Compensation does not include reimbursement for reconstructive therapy, usually because the treatment is not included as part of usual medical methods for joint, tendon, and ligament disabilities.

A typical case was a situation eventually resolved by Kent Pomeroy, M.D. of Scottsdale, Arizona. Dr. Pomeroy is a skilled reconstruction therapist and president of the American Association of Orthopaedic Medicine. The case that follows is true, but the patient's name is changed as are the names of other physicians, insurance companies, and clinics.

Joe Pays for His Own Job-Related Treatment that Works

Joe Paxton, 34, a concrete mason residing in Phoenix, Arizona, enjoyed his outdoors work and the variety associated with different projects given to him by the Smith-Dunn Construction Company of Phoenix. He found masonry to be a creative occupation. His father was a mason, and Joe was able to get his union card as an apprentice mason right after finishing high school. It afforded real freedom and security with a steady and substantial paycheck for such a young fellow. So, at age 26, when he became a journeyman mason, Joe got married and settled into being a family man. He had a good marriage to five-foot, ten-inch Sharon, who eventually became the mother of two curly- haired children, Todd, now seven years old, and Amy, age three.

As a journeyman mason, Joe is strong and heavily muscled on his six-foot, two-inch frame — all 235 pounds of him — solid with no beer-belly. His neck size is 17-1/2, and T-shirts pull tight around his huge, well-defined biceps. He is popular at work, since he can talk sports with the best of them. He enjoys not only watching football and baseball, but he plays them too, mostly on weekends. His bosses like him, as well, because he is dependable, hard working, gives full measure during the eight- hour day, and has a pleasant, enthusiastic personality.

Hard luck hit the concrete mason five years ago when he fell from a slick scaffold suspended ten feet in the air. He landed on his rear end with a jarring crash. His tailbone hurt, and the pains shot into his lumbar spine. He took two weeks off from work and went to a chiropractor for applied kinesiology. X-ray films of his spine revealed that he had a slight compression fracture of the first lumbar vertebra. A soft comfortable back support rest was ordered, and the chiropractic adjustments were directed to maximizing alignment and reducing spasm.

The chiropractic treatments helped Joe, and he returned to heavy labor in just under a fortnight. He continued his chiropractic treatments for three more months and decided to stay with them after his Worker's Compensation case was closed. Depending on how he felt, Joe took the treatments once or twice a month.

On a hot May 1986 morning, the mason was working as a shovel man while a slab was poured for a new high-rise building. The cement truck was putting out the concrete fast, and Joe had to hurry to spread it quickly. He worked like a demon, bent over and twisting to push the concrete around the slab space. Then he felt a pain that took his breath away and literally heard a snap in his low back. Pain shot down the right leg, and he was forced to call for help. Coworkers saw that the man was in pain and in trouble while standing in the wet cement. They ran to his aid.

It took three strong masons to lift him out of the shin-deep ooze. An ambulance transported Joe to St. Alphonse Medical Center where orthopedic and neurological surgeons observed the patient. He exhibited right straight leg raising pain, a decreased Achilles reflex, and other signs of nerve root involvement. A CAT scan, MRI, EMG, and myelogram were performed. These tests revealed irritation of the L4, L5, and S1 nerve roots and L4, L5, S1 bulging vertebral discs. The disc impingements were not quite severe enough for surgery.

Cortisone injections, oral medications, physical therapy, and rest were recommended. The hospital staff carried out the two consultants' instructions. Joe stayed in that hospital for one week. The pain in his leg and back got better, and he found himself walking around and rising from a chair without discomfort about two weeks after he got home.

Joe returned to the chiropractor who administered careful applied kinesiology-directed adjustments to further improve him. Four months after the injury, his orthopedist said that Joe could go back to work, something that the mason was very happy to do. Sitting home watching the "soaps" was not this rugged man's preference.

The first work day involved layering heavy cement blocks that required bending, lifting, stretching and carefully setting the blocks in place. By the job's 4:00 P.M. quitting time, Joe's back was aching in time with his heart. It was a pounding pain, deep into the marrow of his bones. It was obvious to

Sharon that her husband was hurting badly as soon as he stepped through the door of their home. She applied the hydrocollator pack to his body and gave him a massage that she had learned from the chiropractor. Joe took the pain-killer Feldene™ and prescription Tylenol #4™ given to him by the orthopedic surgeon. He went to bed directly. The next morning he felt better, but the twisting and lifting during more hours at work again damaged his back. He called the chiropractor for an emergency visit during the construction company's lunch break.

The application of chiropractic adjustments and electrophysical therapy helped, plus the chiropractor suggested that Joe should resume wearing his soft back support on a continuous basis. He started using this support the next day, even though he felt self conscious — a sign of weakness, he thought, perhaps that he couldn't do his job. Covering the support with clothing prevented fellow workers from spotting it at first, but then they did and repeatedly asked him about his back trouble. By day's end he was again in pain.

Joe consulted his orthopedic surgeon again. After physical and x- ray examination, the doctor told him that inflammation was still present but no further intervertebral disc or nerve damage could be noted on the films. He recommended rest by staying home from work, and he changed the man's pain-killing medication to Naprosyn™.

After taking chiropractic adjustments daily during a six-day break from work, the mason returned to the orthopedist for a progress report. The physician advised that his inflammation was reduced, and he could go back to lifting bricks. Joe did.

This time, deep back aches resumed within four days. More visits to the chiropractor to get temporary relief followed, but Joe felt awful pulling and aching in the back that steadily increased in intensity. He went for more chiropractic adjustments on his lunch hour and then after working hours —

twice daily. The treatments helped but did not hold.

On weekends, instead of playing softball and football with friends as was his regular practice, Joe became a "couch potato" in order to rest his back and be able to return to work Monday morning. He was finding it difficult to get through each eight-hour shift without going off in a corner to rest. A few times the job foreman found him that way and expressed the suspicion that Joe was gold-bricking.

After another consultation, the orthopedic surgeon referred Joe to another neurologist who repeated the EMG and MCI tests. Reports came back that only slight irritations of the lumbar nerve roots existed. This consultant wrote a prescription for Elavil 100™ (100 mg), a new pain-killer, that Joe was to take at bedtime to help the nerve root problem. Each morning thereafter, Joe felt dopey from the pain pill so that the neurologist cut the dosage back to 50 mg.

The Elavil™ produced no particular improvement. It seemed to Joe that his back hurt from any steady use. Rest, chiropractic adjustments, the soft support, medication, and massage all helped a little, but when he returned to work for even part of the day all symptoms of discomfort came back with a vengeance.

One day Joe's sister-in-law, Sonja, telephoned to say that she read an article in the February 1987 issue of *Health Freedom News*, written by a William Faber, D.O. She excitedly told Joe that the article spoke of back pain that persisted and remained unrelieved by traditional methods of treatment but that was resolved by something called "reconstructive therapy". Sonja gave him the telephone number of the Milwaukee Pain Clinic. As it happens, at the moment of Joe Paxton's call, Kent Pomeroy, M.D. of Scottsdale, Arizona was in the Faber clinic.

Ten days later Joe brought his x-ray studies and reports to Dr. Pomeroy who reviewed them and conducted a physical examination of the patient. He had him bend, twist, toe walk, regular walk, and he tapped him, pricked him, and did a dozen tests Joe had gone through before. Then the reconstructive therapist did something more: he put his fingers in the precise areas of the low back that caused the patient sharp pain. Joe was amazed that Dr. Pomeroy could find the exact points where pain was present before Joe identified them. Indeed, Sharon was asked to put her fingers into the weak and torn areas of her husband's superspinous and interspinous ligaments to feel the depressions and mushiness there. No other doctor except, perhaps, the chiropractor had palpated his back in that way.

A drawing of the low back ligaments presented by Dr. Pomeroy showed that when they are strong they work like bridges. No defect between the spines could be felt. However, weakened, shortened, or torn interspinous and superspinous ligaments are different. They possess a sort of hole or divot sunk between the spines. Sharon clearly felt these depressed areas when Dr. Pomeroy explained what to look for. He described why rest, braces, medicines, cortisone, and chiropractics did not resolve Joe's back problem. His spinal column had become unstable from the vertebral discs becoming compressed with tearing and stretching of their ligaments and tendons.

It was obvious that if Joe responded to reconstructive therapeutic injections, he would be stronger than ever. Ligaments would build up and holes or depressions in the spine would disappear. Sharon and Joe wanted Dr. Pomeroy to start reconstructive therapy immediately, and he agreed to do so. Because the ligamentous damage was severe — although never being noticed by the other medical specialists — it could take several months to a year to correct, the doctor said. Still, they would know if the treatment was going to help within the first few treatments.

The beginning series of injection treatments resulted in Joe feeling stiff and sore for two days. When he returned for more a week later, Dr. Pomeroy's probing and palpating caused him less back pain. Joe and Sharon believed that if he obtained more reconstructive treatment, the mason would be back pouring and scooping cement the way he used to do.

The next day, unfortunately, notification came from the Worker's Compensation Insurance Company that Joe must report to industrial physician James Owens, M.D. for an examination in two weeks. Dr. Owens was new to him, so the patient telephoned the insurance company to find out why he was to be examined again. Because it had been eight months since his injury, under existing law the compensation carrier was entitled to have an "independent doctor" check on whether he was faking his pain.

It was then that Joe explained how he had just begun seeing Dr. Pomeroy and with the very first treatment he obtained results that he never had experienced previously. Replying that he was happy Joe was getting assistance, the insurance agent reiterated that it was necessary for him to consult the independent doctor.

Within the next two weeks Joe underwent two additional injection sessions with Dr. Pomeroy. Each injection series had him feel his back to be stronger with greater relief and less pain.

Then, in Dr. Owen's treatment room, Joe went through the same physical examination again, as before. The doctor's report to his insurance carrier would be sent later, the physician/examiner said. No statement of the status of his health was given to Joe at the time of his examination.

One week later the Paxtons found a letter from the insurance carrier in their mailbox. It stated: "Based upon the independent medical examination opinion, it is decided that the healing period for your injuries has ended and no further treatment is necessary. Therefore, it is recommended that you report to work. Any further medical treatment you may choose to have is taken upon your own responsibility." Disability payments were cut off.

Joe and Sharon turned from being happy to sad. They knew he was better but still not strong enough to do the hard work performed by a mason. They decided that Sharon would go back to her job as a waitress on weekends. They would dig into their savings, and on his own Joe would pay for additional reconstructive therapy with Dr. Pomeroy. Fortunately, he needed only two months more of weekly sessions before he was able to return to regular work. While he was working he took more injections because they were bringing him all the way back to good repair — maybe even having a stronger back than before. He went for six months of additional reconstructive therapy.

What Is Wrong with Worker's Compensation Insurance?

Sharon and Joe wondered just what was wrong with the Worker's Compensation Board in that it refused reimbursement for the complete correction of his condition. Why did the "independent doctor and the insurance company that hired him" not allow the patient a resolution of his problem? In response to their questions, Dr. Pomeroy said, "You can't blame them, because they've never been taught reconstructive therapy. Also, they don't really understand your particular back problem. Dr. Owen performed examinations as taught in medical school and residency, but they don't lead to correct conclusions.

"The same situation you face, Joe, repeats itself thousands of times throughout the United States each week with other disabled workers. If the insurance company kept paying your claim and others like it, employers would be unable to afford the insurance premiums," continued Dr. Pomeroy. "You see, millions of employees are hurt on the job, experience joint disabilities, and find no significant aid from traditional medical methods. So they are forced just to cut back on their activities for the balance of their lives. The inevitable result? They lose their jobs, most likely go into bankruptcy, probably get divorced, finally go on Social Security, and eventually receive welfare payments. In this country, job-related injuries are creating a characteristic class of former workers who are disabled and poor. There are about 20 million of them. You are lucky, Joe, you found reconstructive therapy and got your life back just as it was entering that same class of former workers."

Joe thought about this and then said, "But you knew just what to do. How come?"

Dr. Pomeroy smiled and replied, "At one time I did exactly what the independent doctor, your orthopedist, and neurologists did. I followed the methods of traditional allopathic medicine. It's true that I did realize I never really helped joint dysfunction in patients with the methods I was taught in medical school and residency, but those were all that I had to work with. Once I learned about reconstructive therapy, what was once difficult to correct, now has become relatively easy."

Because there has been no previously published medical consumer book like *Pain, Pain Go Away*, the medical profession, the health administrations, insurance companies, and the public at large have overlooked the unsurpassed results of reconstructive therapy. But statistical analysis by computer has not. William Kubitschek, D.O. of San Marcos, California, past president of the American Osteopathic Academy of Sclerotherapy, founding board member of the American Association of Orthopaedic Medicine, and master reconstructive therapist, for years has been expertly applying his science and art to severely injured workers in California.

In his home state, employers may purchase Worker's Compensation Insurance from California or from private insurance companies. The State keeps records of injured workers' progress or lack of it. These records are all on computer. The California officials noted a number of key factors about the San Marcos patients that proved to be striking.

- Dr. Kubitschek's patients returned to work sooner.
- His patients did not relapse.
- The patients did not go on to have costly and often disabling surgery.
- Dr. Kubitschek's patients required fewer disability payments and lower medical costs than those treated by other methods or other doctors.

The California Worker's Compensation Board officials telephoned Carolyn Kubitschek, M.S., the medical office's manager, and explained this to her. Then they referred to the San Marcos reconstruction therapist the most difficult disability cases they could find. These were workers who failed to respond to any other treatment. Again they analyzed the results by computer and came up with impressive numbers. Notable cost savings were shown. The "incurable" patients became productive once again. The result? The State of California asked William Kubitschek, D.O. to become a member of the Board of Directors of the California State Worker's Compensation Panel. He declined, stating that his work is to continue to care for people who simply could not find relief any other way.

Before Taking Reconstructive Therapy, Consider the Following Information

So, have you wondered why you have failed to hear of reconstructive therapy before? We have alluded to a few reasons why this form of complementary medicine may be new to you. There are others, as well. James D. ZeBranek, D.O., a reconstructive therapist located in Garden City,

Michigan, during a 1985 roundtable discussion at the American Association of Orthopaedic Medicine, responded to the question of why this form of complementary medicine may be totally new to you and most other medical consumers. Dr. Zebranek explained:

> Prolotherapy or sclerotherapy — meaning reconstructive therapy — has been taught at what I consider the postgraduate level. It has never been taught in [medical or osteopathic] schools at the undergraduate level — there's been a lack of instructions and a lack of textbook materials. For this reason, familiarity [with the treatment] in the undergraduate level has produced a problem. Consequently most of us, including me, have stumbled into this treatment program by accident. For myself, when I walked into a lecture by Dr. Madson [an expert on circulatory diseases] on varicose vein sclerotherapy in 1975, I said to myself, "Where have I been for all these 25 years of practice? Why didn't I know about this [reconstructive therapy] before?" It's a tool which I could have utilized in helping hundreds and hundreds of people that I have taken care of.

The absence of reconstructive therapy from orthodox medical training is related to differences in medical philosophies. First there is the cornerstone of modern allopathic medicine — testing the effect of disease and drugs on animals and extrapolating the findings to humans. The therapeutics tested, and used, were based on the principle of disease destruction. This requires that a doctor do the opposite of what is necessary to keep the body healthy. Employment of these "opposites" is a practice in contradistinction to the other medical philosophy, the use of medicinal "similars," as developed in homeopathy by Dr. Samuel Hahnemann (1755-1843). Hahnemann wrote:

Each individual case of disease is most surely, radically, rapidly, and permanently annihilated and removed only by a medicine capable of producing in the most similar and complete manner the totality of symptoms, which at the same time are stronger than the disease.[1]

In the United States most of the medicine consumers of health care services receive is centered around the allopathic treatment protocol of opposition to symptoms. Because he or she probably does not understand the homeopathic system of treatment with minute quantities of a remedy that in large doses would produce the symptoms being treated, the traditionalist allopathic physician avoids the remedies of similars.. As we mentioned, allopaths tend to regard homeopaths as "quacks" with their miniscule dosages.

In fact, many of the newest proliferants used in reconstructive therapy are homeopathic remedies injected into joints in tiny doses. In no way could they be accepted by allopathic traditionalists unless the individual doctors became disillusioned with their academic training and became enlightened or opened to the biological or holistic approach of medical practice. That's not readily accomplished after the immense investment of time, money, effort, and shear brain power an M.D. makes in his medical education. It takes an allopathic physician who has done some deep soul-searching to abandon the secure and professionally accepted type of medicine he or she has been taught in school and residency just to provide patients with truer and more effective health care. There is probably a lot of harassment in it from his or her peers, too.

Economic Obstacles to Reconstructive Therapy

Reconstructive therapy is at a disadvantage competing against allopathic products because no organizations have an economic interest in promoting it. Pharmaceutical companies, surgical supply houses, orthopedic surgeons, hospitals, neurologists, pain clinics, and other types of health care professionals spend money to assure active sales of their products and services. Reconstructive therapy tends to disavow the need for such drugs, chemotherapies, and other pharmaceutical agents.

Medical consumers spend huge sums — over $500 billion a year — and produce a good living for probably 20 million who work in the health care industry. In contrast, the application of reconstructive therapy does not produce the large profits furnished by patented drugs, expensive operations, and high technology. While pharmaceutical companies pay for studies in every major university and medical school across the continent, there is no money available to get approval for proliferants by the Food and Drug Administration. The most costly medical innovations (such as heart transplants, artificial ligaments, and other ultra-expensive techniques) usually get all the media attention.

Articles are published in literally thousands of professional journals, books, magazines, and newspapers relating to allopathic breakthroughs. Thousands of sales people call on doctors in their offices and hospitals to inform and help them to use profitable, patented drug products. Reconstructive therapy just does not have any of that money available to reach the medical mainstream. Therefore, someone seeking this outstanding treatment will likely be required to travel far distances to find an experienced practitioner. It's not uncommon for a patient seeking reconstructive therapy to travel several hundred or a thousand miles to receive the treatment from one of the exclusive, skilled, and recommended doctors listed in the Appendix. The permanent, proven correction offered by these remarkably effective injections with proliferants is worth the trip.

Answers to Common Questions
about Reconstructive Therapy

During the course of treatment, questions about reconstructive therapy often arise for patients that should have been answered before the treatment began. Here are the answers to some of these common questions:

How Long Does It Take to Get the Desired Result from Injections with Proliferating Solutions?

Reconstructive therapy is like growing a garden. If the soil is prepared, results can be seen to sprout within a few days to a week after planting. The real harvest comes after repeated cultivation, and it may take a few months to a year. There is no accurate way to predict how long or how many treatments with proliferating solutions are required. Yet, you probably will notice significant improvement in how you feel after about six sessions of injections.

How Often Must the Treatment Be Given?

There is no set frequency of injections. You can go as fast or as slow as is convenient. It does take time for the tissue to grow, however. Usually one week's time permits you to determine what your results will be, although the tissue growth inside ligaments continues for six to eight weeks. Some patients who travel long distances to the reconstructive therapist stay in the doctor's local for a week or two in order to receive intensive therapy. Others arrive for a couple of days of treatment and return when time and financial conditions allow.

Indeed, such effort is called for inasmuch as reconstructive therapy is the most beneficial procedure for the musculoskeletal system known in the history of medicine. If an individual is healthy enough — has a high level of wellness — to obtain noticeable firmness in the treated areas in the first six sessions, each series of injections will build a stronger and more set result for that person. Dr. Faber has never observed a relapse of any joint reconstruction when the patient has undergone maximum reconstruction. Dr. Faber has administered reconstructive therapy to vast numbers of patients with a higher frequency during the past seven years than any other practitioner in the world.

If I've Suffered from a Structural Problem for 50 Years. Can Reconstructive Therapy Help Me?

Yes, joint reconstruction can be effective for damaged discs, joints, cartilage, tendons, ligaments, arthritis, and other difficulties regardless of their duration. Sometimes a limiting factor is your own belief. For example, a famous doctor, or someone at a renowned clinic may say, "You have undergone surgery, so there is nothing more to be done and you need to live with the pain." If you believe this false statement, you'll make it a reality for yourself. In other words, where there is a belief a human will magnify that belief to control and produce the result.

If this Therapy Is So Good, Why Don't You Cite Professional Athletes in this Book Who Have Successfully Undergone Reconstuctive Therapy?

Many professional ball players have been treated with proliferating solutions into their joints, ligaments, and tendons. We are not allowed to reveal the names of these famous people before their contracts run out. The contract of a professional ball player usually contains a clause that requires that the team doctor provide all of the rehabilitative therapy for an injury during play. Those athletes receiving reconstructive therapy must do it quietly and without fanfare; otherwise, their contracts are in jeopardy. Still, you should know that many of the recommended reconstruction therapists on our list have provided proliferant services to famous athletes.

Why Doesn't the Government Financially Support Reconstructive Therapy?

To get the Government's attention on almost any issue, lobbyists who work for a substantial fee are required. This fee often comes from the profits of commercial interests, and no such industry interests exist for reconstructive therapy. But the representatives of our Government should be made aware of advantages of reconstructive therapy. The following is a letter that we suggest you write to your Representative and your Senator:

Dear_____,

The current health insurance cost crisis is not just an administrative problem. It is a fact that the American people (myself among them) feel growing dissatisfaction with the traditional practice of medicine and surgery in this country. It often fails to provide solutions to serious health problems such as chronic joint pain. The health care industry encourages diagnosis and treatment through expensive patented drugs and surgery rather than adjunctive, biological, and/or complementary methods of treatment.

The administration of toxic and unnatural approaches to treatment leads to further illness and its complications. For example, metal joint implants sometimes used to replace parts of an articulation cause cancer, reported the June 12, 1989 issue of *Forbes* magazine.

Did you know that there is a university-proven method to permanently reconstruct tendons, ligaments, and joints called reconstructive therapy which costs less than one-tenth to one-third that of usual methods of treatment?

Did you know that this method has clinically shown itself to be effective for the elimination of back pain, disc herniation, carpal tunnel syndrome, severe arthritis, compression fractures, rotator cuff tears, painful scoliosis, and many other musculoskeletal conditions?

Did you know that some physicians and surgeons state that they "know" about reconstructive therapy and it doesn't work when, in fact, they have never had any training in administering the treatment?

Did you know that there is a book, *Pain, Pain Go Away*, by Faber and Walker that explains and illustrates reconstructive therapy? I have read about reconstructive therapy and am asking you to read about it too. Please take action to see that this treatment becomes the "standard" means of relieving chronic joint pain instead.

President George Bush said during his campaign for the Presidency in 1988 that "in times of crisis private American creativity has always come to the rescue." Please help to make this statement a reality for reconstructive therapy. Please support the study, training, and funding required to establish reconstructive therapy in our country.

Each reconstructive treatment builds health and leads to a joint, tendon, and ligament that is 40 percent stronger than normal. It uses the body's own healing mechanisms. We can not expect to control health care costs or regain our industrial might without improvements in therapy which builds up our bodies. Please come to the aid of your constituents. Thank you!

Yours truly,

How Much Does Reconstructive Therapy Cost?

Taking a series of proliferating injections costs about one-tenth to one-third that of allopathic pharmaceutical and surgical methods. To find out the exact price per visit or per series of injections for the low back, the knee, neck, wrist, ankle, etc., the authors suggest that you telephone the office of your nearest reconstruction therapist.

Should I Telephone or Write My Health Insurance Carrier and Ask If It Covers Reconstructive Therapy?

No, it is best to receive the treatment first and then send in your claim. Usually a physician can provide a proper universal claim form to be sent for receiving reimbursements. Alerting your health insurance company in advance tends to put your claim into audit. Read your insurance policy to learn if it covers injections.

I Want this Reconstructive Therapy, but I Can't Take Shots. Can I Get Results?

You should be careful about saying, "I can't" when you really mean "I won't!" No pills, surgery, or other methods have ever been shown to do what reconstructive therapy does.

My Loved One Desperately Needs Reconstructive Therapy, so How Can I Get Him (Her) to Do It?

You can't get anyone to do anything except to introduce them to this proven method. Perhaps furnish them this book as a gift of love. It's the individual's right to live life as well or as poorly as he or she wishes. A subtle way to draw attention to this treatment is to read aloud the description of a case history or two that is similar to the condition affecting your loved one.

I Have No Reconstruction Therapist within a Few Hundred Miles of Me. What Should I Do?

Travel to wherever the reconstruction therapist is located (see the Appendix) and take the treatment that doctor offers. You can go any time you want to spare the time, money, and inconvenience of travel. Try to take treatment when your healing ability is up to par. Or, perhaps you have a doctor in your own town who is open-minded and tired of never getting his arthritic patients better. You could loan him this book and suggest that he take a preceptorship in reconstruction therapy. Dr. Faber is interested in teaching all practicing clinicians to become masters of this dynamic life-restoring therapy.

My Doctor Is a Skilled Surgeon. If He Obtains the Proliferating Solutions Can He or She Perform the Treatment?

Physicians not specifically preceptor-trained in reconstructive therapy should not attempt to administer it. Diagnostic and treatment skills must be learned first hand. Since the solutions are selected to be irritating, they must be used properly and with caution. Otherwise, less than optimal and even serious complications can take place.

Can I Be Guaranteed a Good Result with Reconstructive Therapy?

No! As in other aspects of living, there are no guarantees. The best chance of getting better is to optimize your diet, take nutrients for immune system boosting, detoxify your bowel, and engage in other aspects of biological therapy. Do all this under the supervision of a biologic or holistic physician, and anticipate that you will receive the kind of physiological results you want from reconstructive therapy.

This book has been written and published strictly for informational purposes, and should not be used as a substitute for

318

advice from your own health professional.

You should in no way consider educational material and/or illustrations found here as replacing consultation with a medical practitioner. However, almost all the facts in this book have come from scientific publications or interviews with informed health care personnel such as medical doctors and osteopathic physicians or their patients who have suffered from chronic joint pain. Most of these patients, eager to share their information about reconstructive therapy that worked well for them, used the authors as their means for communicating with others.

Scientific facts, case histories, and clinical investigations are included in *Pain, Pain Go Away*, but none of the information should be designated as the practice of medicine. The authors of this book and the physicians and patients who contributed as well are merely providing educational material — nothing more. Please take this message as a disavowal of all responsibility by the authors, publisher, and contributors for any health care practice or general information taken from this book and used by you or anyone else.

Footnotes

Chapter Two

1 Vanderschot, Louis. "The American Version of Acupuncture. Prolotherapy: Coming to an Understanding." *American Journal of Acupuncture* 4:4 (Oct.-Dec. 1976) , 309-316.

2 Hippocrates. *The Genuine Works of Hippocrates* [Francis Adams, translator]. (Baltimore: The Williams and Wilkins Co., 1946), pp. 212-214.

3 Valpeau, A.A.L.M. *New Elements of Operative Surgery* [P.S. Townsend, translator]. (New York: Wood, 1847).

4 Gedney, E.H. "Hypermobile Joint." *Osteopathic Profession* 4:9 (1937), 30-31.

5 Schultz, L.W. "A Treatment for Subluxation of the Temporomandibular Joint." *Journal of the American Medical Association* 109 (1937),1032-1035.

6 Shuman, David. "Sclerotherapy." *Osteopathic Annals* 6:12 (December 1978), 10-14.

7 Shuman, David. "Luxation Recurring in Shoulder." *Osteopathic Profession* 8:6 (1941), 11-13.

8 Gedney, E.H. "Disk Syndrome." *Osteopathic Profession* 18:12 (1951), 11-15, 38-46.

9 Hackett, G.S.. Ligament and Tendon Relaxation (Skeletal Disability) Treated by Prolotherapy (Fibro-Osseous Proliferation). (Springfield, Illinois: Charles C. Thomas, 3rd Ed., 1958).

10 Hackett, George S., Huang, T.C., Raftery, Alan, and Theodore J. Dodd. "Back Pain Following Trauma and Disease-- Prolotherapy." *Military Medicine* (July, 1961), 517-525.

11 Hackett, George Stuart. Myoneurovascular Mechanisms. Disease Prevention, Prolotherapy. (Denver: Denver Professional Publishing Co., 1968).

Chapter Three

1 Hackett, George Stuart. Ligament and Tendon Relaxation (Skeletal Disability) Treated by Prolotherapy (Fibro-Osseous Proliferation) (Springfield, IL: Charles C. Thomas, 3rd Ed., 1958), pp. 16-21.

2 Hackett, George S. "Shearing Injury to the Sacroiliac Joint." *The Journal of the International College of Surgeons* 22:6 (Dec. 1954), 631-642.

3 Dosch, Peter. Facts about Neural Therapy According to Huneke [Arthur Lindsay, Translator]. (Heidelberg: Karl F. Haug Publishers, 1985).

4 Hackett, G. S. "Referred Pain from Low Back Ligament Disability." *American Medical Association Archives of Surgery* 73 (Nov. 1956), 878-883.

5 Hackett, G.S. "Prolotherapy for Sciatic from Weak Pelvic Ligaments and Bone Dystrophy." *The Journal of Clinical Medicine* 8 (Dec. 1961), 2301-2316.

6 Howes, R.G. and Isdale, I.C. "The Loose Back: An Unrecognized Syndrome." *Rheumatology and Physical Medicine* 11 (May, 1971), 72-77.

Chapter Four

1 Bronson, Gail. "Beyond the Band-Aid." *Forbes,* (June 1, 1987), pp. 160-161.

2 Hackett, George S. "Low Back Pain." *Industrial Medicine and Surgery* September 1959, pp. 416-419.

3 Liu, Y.K., Tipton, C.M., Matthes, R.D., Bedford, T.G., Maynard, J.A., and W.C. Walmer. "An In Situ Study of the Influence of a Sclerosing Solution in Rabbit Medial Collateral Ligaments and its Junction Strength." *Connective Tissue Research* 11 (1983) pp. 95-102.

4 Ongley, M.J., Dorman, T.A., Eek, B.C., Lundren, D., and R.G. Klein. "Ligament Instability of Knees. A New Approach to Treatment." *Manual Medicine,* 1988.

5 Maynard, J.A., Pedrini, V.A., Pedrini-Mille, A., Romanus, B., and F. Ohlerking. "Morphological and Biochemical Effects of Sodium Morrhuate on Tendons." *Journal of Orthopaedic Research* 3:2 (1985), 236-248.

Chapter Five

1 Hackett, George S. Ligament and Tendon Relaxation Treated by Prolotherapy, 3rd Ed. (Springfield, Mass.: Charles C. Thomas), 1958.

2 Liu, Y.K., et al. "In situ study of sclerosing solution in rabbit knee ligaments." *Connecticut Tissue Research* 11: 95-102, 1983.

Chapter Six

1 Hackett, George S. "Low Back Pain." *Industrial Medicine and Surgery.* September 1959, pp 416-419.

Chapter Seven

1 Ongley, Milne J., Klein, Robert G., Dorman, Thomas A., Eek, Bjorn C., and Hubert, Lawrence J. "A New Approach to the Treatment of Chronic Low Back Pain." *The Lancet* July 18, 1987, pp. 143-146.

2 Hirschberg, G.G., Froetscher, L, and Naeim, F. "Iliolumbar Syndrome as a Common Cause of Low Back Pain: Diagnosis and prognosis." *Archives of Physical Medicine and Rehabilitation* 61:415-419, Sept. 1979.

3 Naeim, Farzan, Froetscher, LeRoy, and Hirschberg, Gerald G. "Treatment of the Chronic Iliolumbar Syndrome by Infiltration of the Iliolumbar Ligament." *Western Journal of Medicine* 136: 372- 374, April 1982.

4 Hackett, George S. Ligament and Tendon Relaxation Treated by Prolotherapy (Springfield, llinois: Charles C. Thomas), 1958.

5 "Soft-Tissue Injections Studied for Back Pain." *Medical World News*, Sept. 28, 1987, pp. 15.

6 Bourdillion, J.F. Spinal Manipulation. 3rd ed. (New York: Appleton-Century Crofts), 1982: 49-122.

7 Million, R., Hall, W., Haavik, Nilsen K., Baker, R.D., Jayson, M.I.V. "Assessment of the Progress of the Back Pain Patient." *Spine* 7:204-212, 1982.

8 Roland, M.R. and Morris, R.M. "A Study of the Natural History of Low Back Pain." *Spine* 8:145-150, 1983.

9 Neson, M.A., Allen, M.B., Clamp, S. E., de Dombal, F.T. "Reliability and Reproducibility of Clinical Findings in Low Back Pain." *Spine* 4:97-101, 1979.

10 Witt, I., Vestergaard, A., Rosenklint, A. "A Comparative Analysis of X-ray Findings of the Lumbar Spine in Patients with and without Lumbar Pain." *Spine* 9:298-300, 1984.

11 Wiesel, S.W., Tsourmas, N., Feffes, H.L. et. al. "A study of Computer-Assisted Tomography. (The Incidence of Positive CAT Scans in an Asymptomatic Group of Patients). *Spine* 9: 549-551, 1984.

12 Roland, M.R. and Morris, R.M. "A Study of the Natural History of Back Pain (Part One: Development of a Reliable and Sensitive Measure of Disability in Low Back Pain) *Spine* 8: 141-144, 1983.

13 Deyo, R.A. "Conservative Therapy for Low Back Pain." *Journal of the American Medical Association* 250: 1057- 1062, 1983.

Chapter Eight

1 Liu, Y.K., Tipton, C.M., Matthes, R.D., Bedford, T.G., Mayunard, J.A., and Walmer, H.C. "An In Situ Study of the Influence of a Sclerosing Solution in Rabbit Medial Collateral Ligaments and Its Junction Strength." *Connective Tissue Research* 11:95-102, 1983

1 Lawrence, J.S. "Disc Degeneration: Its Frequency and Relationship to Symptoms." *Annuals of Rheumatic Diseases* 28:121- 137, 1969.
2 British Association of Physical Medicine. "Pain in the Neck and Arms: A Multicenter Trial of the Effects of Physiotherapy." *British Medical Journal* 1:253-258, 1966.

3 Hult, L. "The Munkfors Investigation." *Acta Orthopedica Scandinavian* Supplement 16:1-76, 1954

4 Hult, L. "Cervical, Dorsal and Lumbar Spinal Syndromes." *Acta Orthopedica Scandinavian Supplement* 17: 1-102, 1954.

5 Brain, W.R. "Discussion on Rupture of the Intervertebral Disc in the Cervical Region." *Procedures of the Royal Society of Medicine* 61:509-516, 1948.

6 Mixter, W. J. and Barr, J.S. "Rupture of the Intervertebral Disc with Involvement of the Spinal Canal." *New England Journal of Medicine* 211:210-215, 1934.

7 Hadler, N.M. "Regional Back Pain." *New England Journal of Medicine* 315:1090-1092, 1986.

8 Deyo, R.A., Diehl, A.K., et al. "How Many Days of Bedrest for Acute Low Back Pain." *New England Journal of Medicine* 315: 1064- 1070, 1986.

9 Bland, John H. "The Cervical Spine: From Anatomy to Clinical Care." *Medical Times*, September 1989, page 28.

10 Kayfetz, Daniel O., Blumenthal, Lester S., Hackett, George S., Hemwall, Gustav A., and Neff, Floyd E. "Whiplash Injury and Other Ligamentous Headache — Its Management with Prolotherapy." *Headache* Vol. III, 1:1-8, April, 1963.

11 Kayfetz, Daniel O. "Occipito-Cervical (Whiplash) Injuries Treated by Prolotherapy." *Medical Trial Technique Quarterly*, June 1963, pp. 9-29.

12 Curd, John G. and Thorne, Roger P. "Diagnosis and Management of Lumbar Disk Disease." *Hospital Practice* Volume 24, 9: 135- 148, Sept. 15, 1989.

13 Blumenthal, Lester S. "Injury to the Cervical Spine as a Cause of Headache." *Postgraduate Medicine* Volume 56, 3:147-153, September 1974.

Chapter Nine

1 Schultz, Louis W. "Twenty Years' Experience in Treating Hypermobility of the Temporomandibular Joints." *American Journal of Surgery* 92: 925-928, December 1956.

2 Schultz, Louis W. "Treatment for Subluxation of the Temporomandibular Joint." *Journal of the American Medical Association* 9: 109-110, 1937.

Chapter Eleven

1 Maynard, J.A., Pedrini-Mille, A., Romanus, B., and Ohlerking, F. "Morphological and Biochemical Effects of Sodium Morrhuate on Tendon." *Journal of Orthopaedic Research* 3: 236-248, 1985.

2 Ongley, Milne J., Dorman, Thomas A., Eek, Bjorn C., Lundgren, David, and Klein, Robert G. "Ligament Instability of Knees: A New Approach to Treatment." *Manual Medicine* 3: 152-154, 1988.

3 Daniel, D.M., Malcolm, L.L., Losse, G., Stone, M.L., Sachs, R., and Burks, R. "Instrument Measurement of Anterior Laxity of the Knee." *Journal of Bone and Joint Surgery* 67: 720-725, 1985.

4 Highgenboten, C.L. "The Reliability of the Genucom Knee Analysis System." The Second European Congress of Knee Surgery and Arthroscopy held in Basle, Switzerland, Sept. 29, 1986.

5 Ongley, M.J., Klein, R.G., Dorman, T.A., Eek, B.C., and Huber, L. "A New Approach to the Treatment of Chronic Low Back Pain." *Lancet II*: 143-146, 1987.

6 Keene, James S. "Diagnosis of Undetected Knee Injuries." *Post Graduate Medicine* Vol. 85, 4: 153-163, March 1989.

Chapter Twelve

1 It happens that this book's coauthor, Morton Walker, D.P.M. of Stamford, Connecticut, competed against Dr. Bronston that year and surpassed him by winning the Bronze Medal and a cash award for original clinical research and writing on fungus diseases of the feet. Dr. Walker went on to win ten such research, writing, and exhibits awards from the American Podiatry Association — more than any other practicing podiatrist ever has done. His recognitions and plaudits from colleagues included their bestowing on him multiple Silver Medals and Bronze Medals, plus the Association's highest research and writing award, the William J. Stickel Fiftieth Anniversary Gold Medal (in 1962) for Research and Writing in Podiatric Medicine. These ten awards plus nine other medical journalism awards bestowed on him by The Journal of Current Podiatric Medicine were accumulated in just ten years, since Dr. Walker left the practice of podiatric medicine in 1969 to become a fulltime, professional, freelance medical journalist specializing in the writing of books and articles about holistic or biological medicine, orthomolecular nutrition, and alternative or complementary methods of healing.

2 Bronston, Gordon J. "The Strengthening of Chronically Stained Ankle Ligaments with Injections of Sodium Psylliate." *Journal of the American Podiatry Association* Volume 48, 11: 511-516, November, 1958.

Chapter Thirteen

1 "Orthopedic Surgeons Ponder: How Best to Secure Artificial Hip Prostheses?" *JAMA*, Volume 258, 2:173, July 10, 1987.

2 Hackett, George S. and Huang, T.C. "Prolotherapy for Sciatica from Weak Pelvic Ligaments and Bone Dystrophy." *Clinical Medicine* Volume 8, number 12, December 1961.

3 Walmer, Harold C. "A Chronic Dislocated Hip Prosthesis Successfully Treated by Sclerotherpy: A Case Report." *Pennsylvania Osteopathic Medical Association Journal*, Volume 26, 3: 8 & 9, Summer 1982.

4 Faber, William J. "Carpal Tunnel Syndrome (CTS) an Alternative View and Treatment Approach." *The Journal of Neurological and Orthopaedic Medicine and Surgery* Volume 11, Issue 1, April 1990 (in press).

5 Spinner, R.J., Bachman, J.W., Amadio, P.C. "The Many Faces of Carpal Tunnel Syndrome." *Mayo Clinic Proceedings* 64:829-836, July 1989.

6 Masear, V."., Hayes, J.M., Hyde, A.G. "An Industrial Cause of Carpal Tunnel Syndrome." *American Journal of Hand Surgery* 11: 222-227, 1986.

Chapter Fourteen

1 Kent, James M. "Safe, Useful Manipulative Techniques." *Patient Care*, August 15, 1984, pp. 137-189.

2 Edsall, Robert L. RManipulation: A Tool for Your Practice?" *Patient Care*, May 15, 1984, pp. 16-97.

3 Caillet, Rene, Understand Your Backache: A Guide to Prevention, Treatment, and Relief (Philadelphia: F.A. Davis Co., 1984), p. 138.

4 Ibid. p. 139.

Chapter Fifteen

1 Empting-Koschorke, L.D., Hendler, Nelson, Kolodny, A. Lewis, and Kraus, Hans. "When pain is intractable." *Patient Care* June 15, 1989, pp 407-125.

Chapter Sixteen

1 "Chronic Pain: Sizing Up the Team Approach." *Medical World News*, August 28, 1989, pp. 43-48.

2 Nelson, D.A. "Dangers from methylprednisolone acetate therapy by intraspinal injection." *Archives of Neurology* 45 (7): 804-806, July 1988.

3 Dickey, W. and Patterson, V. "Bilateral Achilles tendon rupture simulating peripheral neuropathy: unusual complication of steroid therapy." *Journal of R. Soc. Medicine* 80(6): 386-387, June 1987.

4 Mitova, M., Maslan, J., Jezova, D., and Svobodova, J. "The effect of Kenalog administration into the joints or tendons of rat extremities on the vital organs." *Acta Chir Orthop Traumatol Cech* 54(6): 499-507, Dec. 1987.Huon, S.K., Wang, C.W., Hsu, W.Y., and Chung, M.T.

5 Huon, S.K., Wang, C.W., Hsu, W.Y., and Chung, M.T. "Ruptured achilles tendon — a case report and literature review. *Chung Hua I Hsueh Tsa Chih* 39(4): 291-296, April 1987.

6 Chiarelli, G. and Del-Borrello, E. "Spontaneous and iatrogenic subcutaneous rupture of the tendons of the hand: experimental study." *Chir Organi Mov* 71(2): 151-157, Apr.-June 1986.

7 Alexeeff, M. "Ligamentum patellae rupture following local steroid injection." *Australian-New Zealand Journal of Surgery* 56(9): 681-683, September 1986.

8 Price, A.E., Evanski, P.M., and Waugh, T.". "Bilateral simultaneous Achilles tendon ruptures. A case report and review of the literature." *Clinical Orthopedics* 213: 249-250, Dec. 1986.

9 Kredskild, O. and Kodal, T. "Rupture of the patellar ligament after steroid infiltration." *Ugeskr Laeger* 149(5): 300-301, January 26, 1987.

10 Saether, J. and Srensen, J. "Avulsion of the Achilles tendon after a single steroid injection." *Ugeskr Laeger* 149(5): 299-300, January 26, 1987.

Chapter Seventeen

1 Hahnemann, Samuel. The Organon of Medicine, translated with Preface by William Boericke (Philadelphia: Boericke and Tafel, 1922).

Appendix

Physicians Administering Reconstructive Therapy

Alabama
Gus J. Prosch, Jr., M. D.
759 Valley Street
Birmingham, AL 35226

Alaska
Robert Rowan, M. D.*
615 East 82nd Avenue
Suite 300
Anchorage, AK 99518

Arizona
Ellis Browning, M.D.
1150 West 24th Street
Suite F
Yuma, AZ 85258

Kent Pomeroy, M.D.
9755 North 90th Street
Suite A-205
Scottsdale, AZ 85258

California
Thomas A. Dorman, M.D.
1041 Murray Avenue
San Luis Obispo, CA 93401

Bjorn Eek, M.D.
2927 De La Vina, Ste. D
Santa Barbara, CA 93105

Robert G. Klein, M.D.
2927 De La Vina, Ste. D
Santa Barbara, CA 93105

William Kubitschek, D. O.
1194 Calle Maria
San Marcos, CA 92069

Andrew Kulik, D. O.
218D Garnet Ave, Ste. 1B
San Diego, CA 92109

Craig Miller, M. D.
212 N. San Mateo Dr.
San Mateo, CA 94401

Harish Porecha, M. D.*
1401 Stands Ct.
Modesto, CA 95355

Felix Prakasam, M. D.*
415 Brookside Ave.
Redlands, CA 92373

Bharati Shah, M. D.*
190 E. Latham Ave.
Hemet, CA 92543

Florida
Hana T. Chaim, D.O.*
595 W. Granada Blvd.
Suite D
Ormond Beach, FL 32174

Alfred S. Massam, M. D.*
P.O. Box 1328
528 W. Main
Wauchula, FL 33873

Georgia
Glynn Taunton, D. O.*
300 Medical Court
Oglethorpe, GA 31068

Hawaii
Joseph A. Brock, M. D.*
(retired)
1380 Lusitana, Suite 905
Honolulu, HI 96813

Indiana
David Dietz, M. D.*
2810 Ethel
Muncie, IN 47304

Iowa
David P. Nebbeling, D.O.*
622 E. 38th
Davenport, IA 52807

Kansas
Arthur Dowell, M. D.*
501 Mur-len
Olathe, KS 66062

Michigan
Marvin D. Penwell, D. O.*
319 S. Bridge St.
Linden, MI 48451

326

Missouri

Edward McDonagh, D. O.*
2800 A. Kendallwood
Parkway
Gladstone, MO 64199

New Jersey

Herbert Fichman, D.O.
Box 642, R. D. #2
Granttown Road
Turnersville, NJ 08012

New York

Chris Calapa, D.O.*
18 E. 53rd Street
New York, NY 10022

Alfredo Castillo, M.D.*
126 Wieland Avenue
Staten Island, NY 10309

Donald Fraser, M.D.
5147 Lewiston Road
Lewiston, NY 14092

North Dakota

Brian E. Briggs, M.D.*
718 6th Street S.W.
Minot, ND 58701

Ohio

L. Terry Chappell, M.D.*
122 Thurman Street
Bluffton, OH 45817

Douglas C. Weeks, M.D.*
24700 Center Ridge Rd.
Cleveland, OH 44131

Oklahoma

Crafton James, D.O.*
3750 So. Peoria Ave.
Tulsa, OK 74104

Pennsylvania

Rodney Chase, D.O.
1343 Easton Avenue
Bethlehem, PA 18018

Jack Smith, D.O.
331 Pittsburgh Road
Butler, PA 16001

Harold Walmer, D.O.
(retired)
50 North Market Street
Elizabethtown, PA 17022

Tennessee

James A. Carlson, D.O.
509 North Cedar Bluff Rd.
Knoxville, TN 37923

Texas

John Sessions, D.O.
1609 South Margaret
Kirbyville, TX 75956

John Parks Trowbridge,
M.D.*
9816 Memorial Blvd.
Suite 205
Humble, TX 77338

Anthony Valdez, M.D.*
1501 Arizona, Bldg.10
El Paso, TX 79902

Wisconsin

William J. Faber, D.O.
6529 West Fond du Lac Ave.
Milwaukee, WI 53218

Australia

Heather Bassett, M.B.*
91 Donnison St.
Gosford, Australia 2250

Canada

Jean R. Aubrey, M.D.
65-B Queen Street
P.O. Box 2230
Sturgeon Falls,
Ontario P0H 2G0

Yvon Bordueau, M.D.
2555 St. Joseph Boulevard
Orleans, Ontario K1C 1S6

Real Dumontier, M.D.
C.P. 189 Spacefield
Orleans, Ontario J0X 1W0

Jean Paul Ouellette, M.D.
2555 St. Joseph Boulevard
Orleans, Ontario K1C 1S6

Maurice Proulx, M.D.
1 Westmont Square, #745
Westmont, Montreal,
Quebec H3Z 2P9

South Africa

C.J. Thiart, M. D.*
48 Villa Street
Clydesdale
Pretoria 0002

* trained by William J. Faber, D.O. Please send a self-addressed stamped legal-size envelope to Dr. Faber for an updated list of physicians newly trained in your area.

For information regarding the use of this treatment for animals, send a self-addressed stamped legal-size envelope to: American Holistic Veterinary Medical Association, 2214 Old Emmorton Road, Bel Air, MD 21014.

INDEX

GLOSSARY

ABOLISH - get rid of

ABSCESS - a collection of pus forming in a tissue space as a result of infection

ABSORB - suck or draw up

ACHIEVE - succeed or accomplish

ACHILLES TENDON - the tendon of the gastrocnemius and soleus muscle

ACUPUNCTURE - puncture of the skin or tissue by one or more needles

ADIPOSE - obese: fat in connective tissue

ADRENAL - Endocrine glands located above the kidneys

AGGRAVATE - make worse

ALLOCATE -distribute in shares

ALLOPATHIC - a Galenic treatment by drugs which produce phenomena different from those of the disease treated

AMALGAM - a combination of mercury, tin and silver used for filling of caries in the teeth

AMENABLE - something done which is able to make up for injury; able to be controlled or influenced

AMORPHOUS - formless; non crystalline

ANALGESIC - relieving pain; remedy that relieves pain

ANCILLARY - subordinate that serves as an aid

ANKYLOSING - spondylitis; joining of the bones forming an articulation, resulting in a stiff joint and inflammation of one or more vertebrae

ANTERIOR - before or in front of

ANTIDOTE - an agent preventing or counteracting the action of poison

ANTIDROMIC - pertaining to impulses passing in the opposite direction to the normal

APOPHYSEAL - growth, relating to an apophysis, a bony protuberance which was never during its development separated from the bone by cartilage

ARMAMENTARIUM - outfit of medicine or instruments

ARTHROPATHOLOGY - joint pathology

ARTERIOSCLEROSIS - chronic morbid condition of the vertical walls, characterized by a thickening and decreasing elasticity of the walls and narrowing of the lumen

ARTICULAR - divided into joints; distinct or clear

ARTICULATION - joining or being joined

ASYMMETRY - absence of symmetry, unequal sides

ATLAS - first cervical vertebrae

ATROPHY - diminution in volume or abnormal smallness of cells, tissues or organs resulting from developmental or nutritional disturbance

AVASCULAR - bloodless

BIO-CHEMISTRY - the chemistry of living tissues

BUCKS EXTENSION - an apparatus consisting of a weight and pulley for applying extension to a limb

C.A.T. SCAN - computerized axial tomography - specialized computer x-ray

CANDIDA - yeast infection

CANTILEVER - a large bracket projecting from a wall

CAPITULUM - the bulb of a hair; small rounded prominence of a bone; the rounded eminence at the lower end of the humerus

CAPSULAR - relating to a capsule

CARDIOVASCULAR - relating to heart and blood vessels

CARTILAGE - gristle; a tissue forming the main part of the embryonic skeleton in vertebrae, becoming in nearly all vertebrae converted into bone and hyaline which consists of an avascular intercellular tissue with cells interspersed

CARTILAGINOUS - having the nature of cartilage

CATWALK - narrow elevated walkway

CAUTERIZING - burning with a cautery, or the process of applying one

CAUTERY - an instrument for destroying tissue by burning

CELLULAR HYPERPLASIA - an increase in the size of a tissue or an organ, due to an increase in the number of cells

CERVICAL SPINE - the neck and first part of the spinal cord

CHEMOTHERAPY - prevention or treatment of disease by chemical substances which are effective against the pathogenic organism or disease

CHYMOPAPAIN INJECTION - enzyme injection to dissolve tissue

331

CLAVICLE - collar bone
CLINICAL - seen in patient examination
COAGULATE - the conversion to a gel state of a liquid; to clot
COLLABORATE - work together
COLLAGEN - a protein structural tissue
COLLATERAL - accompanying blood circulation through anastomosing vessels
COMPONENT - ingredient in a mixture
COMPRESSION - forcing together, often resulting in smaller structure
COMPRESSION FRACTURE - compression forcing breakage, especially of a bone
CONDYLOTOMY - division of a condyle; extra-articular osteotomy
CONDYLES - rounded articular eminence
CONGENITAL - actually or potentially present at birth
CONGENITALLY ANOMALOUS - actually or potentially present at birth, resulting in abnormality
CONJECTURE - arrive at or guess
CONTIGUOUS - in actual contact
CONTRAINDICATE - make a particular method of treatment inadvisable or forbidden
CONTRAINDICATION - anything forbidding a particular method of treatment
CONVALESCENCE - period of recovery from an illness
CORACOACROMIAL - relating to both coracoid process and acromion of the shoulder
CORACOID SYNDROME - shaped like crow's beak
CORTICOSTEROID - generic term for steroid substance found in the adrenal cortex
CRANIUM - the skull of a vertebrate animal
CREPITATION - the grating or crackling sound produced by the friction of two rough surfaces, such as the free ends of a fractured bone in an osteoarthritic joint, or in dry pleurisy
CRUCIATE - cross shaped; ligament within knee
CYLINDRICAL - relating to or shaped like a cylinder
D. C. - Doctor of Chiropractic
D. O. - Doctor of Osteopathy
DEBILITATE - weaken
DECELERATE - reduce speed
DEFECATE - excrete waste matter
DEFERENCE - putting off to a future time; yielding to the opinion of another
DELETERIOUS - harmful
DEMYELINATING - applied to nerve fibers which have lost their protective sheaths
DEPICT - picture in words, describe
DETOX - the removal of toxic properties or effects
DEXTROSE - glucose, a sugar solution commonly used in intravenous formulas
DIAGNOSTIC - the art or practice of diagnosis
DIATHERMY - therapy applied to body through radiant heat
DILATE - enlarge, expand
DILATION - enlargement, spreading apart or expansion
DISC - circular plate or surface
DISCREPANCY - lack of agreement
DISINTEGRATE - separate into parts
DISSECTION - cutting of parts of the body along natural lines of cleavage
DISSIPATED - having dispersed matter
DISTAL END - farthest from the center or point of attachment
DORSAL - pertaining to the posterior part of an organ
DUPUYTREN'S CONTRACTION - contraction of the palmar fascia of the hand
DYSFUNCTION - impaired function, especially qualitatively abnormal function
EFFICACY - power to produce effects or intended results
EFFUSION - a pouring out
ELASTICITY - the property of a body to resist a deforming force by returning to its original shape after discontinuation of that force
ELECTRON - a particle of negative electric charge
ELONGATE - make or become large
EMPATHY - close emotional communion between two persons, especially that believed to develop between an infant and its mother
ENCROACH - advance beyond the usual limits or intrude upon another's space
ENDORPHINS - secretions in the brain which have a pain-relieving affect
EPIDEMIOLOGY - the branch of medicine that investigates causes and control of epidemics
EPIDURAL - an injection under the dural covering of the spine

EPISODIC - having the nature of an episode

EROSION - scraping away or curetting

EXACERBATE - increase the severity of a disease

EXCRUCIATING - greatly painful

EXPONENT - a person who sets forth or explains principals or methods

EXTEROCEPTIVE - pertaining to stimuli upon an exteroceptor; a sense organ responding to stimuli arising outside the body

EXTREMITIES - body limbs (hands or feet)

EXTRINSIC - external; originating on the outside

FACET - a small planed surface on which spinal joints move

FALLACIOUS - erroneous; tending to mislead or deceive

FASCITIS - inflammation of a fascia (fibro-elastic tissue ensheathing muscles)

FELDENKRAIS TECHNIQUE - a slow movement technique to increase range of motion

FEMORAL JOINT - thigh bone joint

FIBRO-OSSEOUS JUNCTION - the place where ligaments and tendons originate and attach to the bones

FIBROBLAST - a mesenchymal cell giving production of connective tissue

FLATULENCE - the presence of abnormal amounts of gas in the bowels

FOCAL INFECTION - a localized infection

FUNCTIONAL STIMULATOR - relating to the special action of an organ

FUSE - melt or join together

GANGLION - a mass of nerve cells serving as a center from which nerve impulses are transmitted

GLENOID - having or resembling a shallow cavity or socket of shoulder

GLUTEAL - relating to the buttocks

GLYCERINE - a syrupy liquid used as solvent, skin lotion, etc.

GOUTY ARTHRITIS - a hereditary form of arthritis resulting from excessive uric acid accumulation in joints

GRANULATION - any small, soft, reddish nodules mainly consisting of capillaries, histocytes and lymphocytes, forming in the repair of a wound or ulcer

HARBOR - provide a place of refuge or safety

HERNIATED - having a hernia

HIGH AMPLITUDE - the extreme position of a vibratory body (e.g. pendulum) away from the mean

HUMERUS - bone of the upper arm

HYPERMOBILITY - excessive increase in movement

HYPERPLASIA - an increase in the size of a tissue or an organ due to an increase in the number of cells

HYPERTHERMIA - rise of body temperature not due to bacterial invasion

HYPERTONIC - abnormal increase of muscular tonicity or high osmotic pressure

HYPERTROPHY - a state of increased development in size of muscles or tissue

ILIOLUMBAR - pertaining to the back

ILIUM - the flank bone of the pelvis

IMMUNOSUPPRESSION - deliberate inhibition of the normal immune response, especially to permit successful organ grafting, by medical or physical means

IMPINGEMENT - encroachment upon the rights of another

INELASTIC - not elastic

INFILTRATION - entrance into cells or intercellular spaces by some abnormal substance

INFUSION - the process of extracting the active principles of a vegetable substance by water that has been heated to the boiling point ;introduction of solution into the body, specifically into a vein

INHIBIT - restrain or suppress

INORDINATE - disorderly

INTERNIST - doctor who specializes in Internal Medicine

INTERSPINAL - between the vertebrae spines

INTERVERTEBRAL - between the vertebrae

INTERVERTEBRAL FORAMINA - situated between the vertebrae forming a hole or window

INTESTINAL RUPTURE - tearing or bursting of intestine

INTOLERANCE - inability to tolerate a particular drug

INTRALIGAMENTOUS - situated within or in folds of a ligament

INTRINSIC - situated within

LATERAL - at or belonging to the side

LATERAL CURVATURE - at or belonging to the side away from the central plane

LAXITY - looseness

LIDOCAINE - a local anesthetic

LIGAMENT - a band of tough tissue connecting bones or holding organs in place

LOIN - the lateral and posterior region of the trunk between the lower ribs and the iliac crest

LORDOSIS - abnormal curvature of the spine forward

LUMBAR LORDOSIS - abnormal curvature of the lumbar spine forward

LUMBOSACRAL - relating to the lumbar vertebrae and sacrum

LYMPHATIC - relating to or characterized by lymph

M. D. - doctor of Medicine

MALAISE - general feeling of being unwell

MALOCCLUSION - the occlusion of teeth not in their anatomical site; misaligned bite

MANDIBLE - lower jaw

MANIFEST - to make clear or evident, reveal

MANIPULATION - handling; the treatment of diseases or injuries of the joints, ligaments and bones etc., mainly by the performance of certain passive movements of the injured part

MARATHON - any long distance or endurance contest

MATRIX - a mass of connective tissue in which something is embedded

MENISCECTOMY - removal of intra-articular cartilagineous meniscus, usually applied to the knee joint

MENISCUS - an interarticular fibro-cartilagineous disc

METABOLIC DISTURBANCE - the sign of physical and chemical changes in a living body

METHYLPREDNISOLONE ACETATE - an adrenal corticosteroid

MICRO ADHESIONS - small areas of tissue stuck together

MINUSCULE - very tiny; minute

MISDIAGNOSIS - wrong diagnosis

MODULATE - to regulate, adjust or adapt to the proper degree

MORPHOLOGY - the whole form or structure of an organism

MOTOR WEAKNESS - difficulty in moving or walking

MULTIFACTORIAL - pertaining to many facts

MUSCULAR SPLINTING - stiffening of the muscles to prevent motion of a joint

MUSCULOSKELETAL - muscle which is connected to a bone; mainly striated

MYELOGRAM - radiological examination of the spinal cord after introduction of an x-ray dye

NAPROSYN - an anti-inflammatory drug for arthritis

NEMESIS - an opponent for which victory seems inevitable

NEUROTRANSMITTER - a substance that transmits or inhibits nerve impulses from nerve cell to another cell

NEURITIS - pain and loss of normal function caused by lesion of a peripheral nerve

NEUROCHEMISTRY - relating to chemistry of nerves

NEUROPATHY - any disease of the nervous system

NEUROSURGEON - a specialist in surgery on the nervous system

NEUROSURGERY - the surgery of the central and peripheral nervous system

NODE - a knot or excrescence

NYSTAGMUS - involuntary rhythmic movement of the eyeballs, usually side to side

OBLIQUE - slanting; inclined; not direct

OBLITERATION - entire closure of a lumen or cavity

OCCIPITOCERVICAL - relating to occiput and neck

OSSEOUS - bony

OSTEOPHYTE - a small localized cortical or subcortical deposit of bone from the periosteum

OSTEOPOROSIS - local or generalized bone atrophy which is characterized by a loss of osseous tissue without any change in the shape of the connected bones

PALPATE - examine by touch

PANACEA - a remedy alleged to cure every disease

PARADOX - a statement that is seemingly ridiculous or contradictory and yet is perhaps true

PASSIVE - not active

PASSIVE CONGESTION - congestion due to obstruction or venous flow

PECTORAL - concerning the chest

PELVIC - relating to pelvis

PERCEPTION - mental grasp of objects, qualities, etc., by means of the senses; awareness

PERIFORNIC - pearshaped; a small bone

situated on the anterior and inner portion of the carpus

PERIPHERAL NERVE - any motor, sensory or mixed nerve connecting the end; organs - receptor or effector, with the spinal cord or brain, excluding the autonomic nerve and usually excluding the cranial nerves

PERMEATE -pass into and affect every part of a thing

PERSONA - outer personality or facade presented to others

PHARMACEUTICAL - chemistry of substances in and related to the practice of pharmacy

PHARMACOLOGICAL SENSORY - the science of the properties of drugs

PHARYNX - throat or gullet

PHENOL - solid melting at 43 degrees C., obtained from the distillation of cool tar, having a characteristic odor, and irritating because of its rapid corrosive action on tissues

PHYSIOLOGICAL PROCESSES - the science of functions of a living organism and its parts

PILGRIMAGE - any long journey to a place of historical interest

PINNACLE - a pointed formation; the top point

PLACEBO - a medicine or treatment given to humor the patient; a sugar pill

PLATELETS - small cells which have a function in blood clotting

POLARITY THERAPY - a therapy given with the hands to balance body energy

POLYMYALGIA - pain, in dry pleurisy, in a number of muscles

POPLITEAL - relating to the part of the leg behind the knee

POST MENOPAUSAL - after menopause

POSTERIOR - placed behind

PRECEPTORSHIP - teaching program in which student studies with teacher while doing actual work

PREDISPOSED - susceptible to a disease or condition

PROGNOSIS - forecast of the probable duration, course and termination of disease

PROJECTION - something that sticks out or protrudes

PROLAPSE - the falling forward or downward of a part

PROLES - production of fibrous tissue

PROLIFERATING - multiplying; characterized by the formation of new tissue

PROLIFERATION - reproduction rapidly and repeatedly of new parts, as by cell division

PROLIFERATIVE THERAPY - treatment given to cause formation of new tissue

PRONATION - rotation of forearm, hand or foot so palm or sole faces downward

PROSTAGLANDIN - any of a group of hormone-like fatty acids found throughout the body that affect blood pressure, metabolism and body temperature

PROTOCOL - a set of rules for conduct or a specific method of treatment

PROXIMAL - situated nearest to the center of the body

PSYCHOLOGICAL - affecting the mind

PUPILLARY - relating to the pupil of the eye

PURINE - heterocyclic compound

PYROGEN FREE - not containing any agent which could cause infection or fever

RADIATING - diverging from a common center

RADIOLOGICAL - relating to radiology, x-rays

RANDOMIZED - given at random

RECEPTOR - any group of substances found on the surface of a cell

REFLEX SYMPATHETIC DYSTROPHY - a complex nerve disorder resulting in contracture, pain and muscle wasting

REPETITIVE -repeating the same motion

REPRODUCE -bring forth offspring

RETICULAR FIBERS - net-like structure

RHEUMATOID - characterized by painful inflammation and stiffness of joints

RHEUMATOLOGIST - one who treats rheumatic diseases

RHOMBOID - shaped like a rhomb, diamond-shaped; R. fascia - the fourth ventricle of the brain

RHYTHMIC LINEAR STRETCHING - rhythmic stretching in a straight line

ROENTGENOLOGY - study and use of x-rays in diagnosis and treatment of disease

SACRAL - relating to sacrum

SACRAL TORSION - twisting of the sacrum

SACROILIAC - relating to the sacrum and ilium

SACROSPINALIS - erector spinal muscle

SADDLE SENSORY - nerve dysfunction in pelvis in the distribution of a saddle

SALINE - salty solution

SALIVATION - excessive flow of saliva

SCARIFICATION - making of a quantity of small superficial incisions in the skin

SCHIZOPHRENIA - a chronic progressive mental disorder usually starting in early adult life characterized by a distortion of reality, delusions and hallucinations

SCLEROTHERAPY - reconstructive therapy; a method of inducing irritants by injection to cause production of tissue

SEDENTARY - fixed to one spot

SEMILUNAR - crescent moon-shaped

SHINGLES - an acute, inflammatory, painful disease, showing grouped cutaneous vesicles along the course of the cutaneous nerves, generally the cutaneous branches of the intercostal nerves

SOMATIC - relating to the body and the body framework

SPECIFICITY THEORY - the condition of being specific; a medicine with a distinct influence on a particular disease

SPHERICAL - relating to a sphere; round

SPHINCTER - muscle surrounding and serving to close a body orifice

SPINOUS - like a spine or thorn in form

SPINOUS PROCESS - the backward-directed process arising from the junction of the spinal laminae

SPUR - any sharp point or projection

STABILIZE - keep in a fixed position

STERNOMASTOID - a muscle, relating to the sternum and mastoid process of the temporal bone

STIMULATE - excite; quicken; promote functional activity

SUBARACHNOID - located beneath the arachnoid membrane of the brain and spinal cord

SUBCLINICAL - term applied to an infection or disease which is so mild that it does not give rise to clinical signs and symptoms which would allow for a diagnosis

SUBCUTANEOUS - lying or occurring beneath the skin

SUBJECTIVE - produced by the mind or a particular state of mind

SUBLUXATION - a sprain or incomplete dislocation

SUBOCCIPITAL - beneath the occiput or back part of the head

SUBSCAPULAR - beneath the scapula

SUPERFICIAL FLEXOR - a muscle that bends a limb or a part

SUPRASPINATUS MUSCLE - the muscle which moves shoulder joint, raises arm and adducts arm

SYMPTOMATOLOGY - the study of symptoms

TENS UNIT - unit attached to spine for self-regulation of pain by electrical current

T.M.J. - temporomandibular; lower jaw joint

TALOCALCANEAL - relating to the talus and the calcaneum bones of ankle

TENDINOUS - relating to tendon

TENOSYNOVITIS - inflammation of a tendon and its sheath

TERMINAL - the final stages of fatal disease

THORACIC - relating to the chest

TINNITUS - a ringing or roaring in the ear

TONUS - tone

TOXICITY - the quality of being poisonous

TRANSIENT - not enduring or permanent

TRANSVERSELY ELLIPTICAL - oval-shaped side to side

TRAPEZIUM - the first bone of the second row of carpal bones

TRAPEZIUS - inserted into the clavicle, spine or scapula, and acromion; rotates the scapula

TRIGEMINAL NEURALGIA - pain in the face about the fifth cranial nerve

TRUNK - the body of a human being, not including head or limbs

URIC ACID - a product of nuclein metabolism found in blood and urine

URINARY TRACT - the tract that carries away fluid secreted by the kidneys, passing into the bladder and finally discharged by the urethra

VASOMOTOR - of, relating to, or being nerves regulating the size in diameter of blood vessels

VERTIGO - lack of equilibrium; dizziness

VESICLE - a skin blister such as herpes or chickenpox

VEXATION - cause of annoyance

VIRAL - caused by virus

WBC - white blood cell